W9-AMU-710

TONE YOUR TUMMY TYPE

TONE YOUR TUMMY TYPE

FLATTEN YOUR BELLY AND SHRINK YOUR WAIST IN 4 WEEKS

DENISE AUSTIN

Star of *The Daily Workout*, *Lifetime*.

Notice

This book is intended as a reference volume only, not as a medical manual. The information given here is designed to help you make informed decisions about your health, diet, fitness, and exercise program. It is not intended as a substitute for professional fitness and medical advice. If you suspect that you have a medical problem, we urge you to seek competent medical help. As with all exercise programs, you should seek your doctor's approval before you begin.

Mention of specific companies, organizations, or authorities in this book does not imply endorsement by the publisher, nor does mention of specific companies, organizations, or authorities imply that they endorse this book.

Internet addresses and telephone numbers given in this book were accurate at the time it went to press.

© 2007 by Denise Austin

All rights reserved. No part of this publication may be reproduced or transmitted in any form or by any means, electronic or mechanical, including photocopying, recording, or any other information storage and retrieval system, without the written permission of the publisher.

Rodale books may be purchased for business or promotional use or for special sales. For information, please write to: Special Markets Department, Rodale Inc., 733 Third Avenue, New York, NY 10017.

Printed in the United States of America
Rodale Inc. makes every effort to use acid-free ♾, recycled paper ♻.

All interior photographs by Mitch Mandel/Rodale Images with the exception of the following:
page v, courtesy of the author; pages 1, 29, 81, and 203 © Hilmar.
Book design by Tara Long

Library of Congress Cataloging-in-Publication Data

Austin, Denise.
    Tone your tummy type : flatten your belly and shrink your waist in 4 weeks / by Denise Austin.
        p.   cm.
    Includes index.
    ISBN-13 978–1–59486–472–8 hardcover
    ISBN-10 1–59486–472–1 hardcover
    ISBN-13 978–1–59486–814–6 paperback
    ISBN-10 1–59486–814–X paperback
    1. Reducing exercises.   2. Weight loss.   3. Abdominal exercises.   I. Title.
    RA781.6.A894 2006
    613.7'12—dc22   2006029363

Distributed to the trade by Macmillan

    4 6 8 10 9 7 5 3   hardcover
2 4 6 8 10 9 7 5 3 1   paperback

RODALE
LIVE YOUR WHOLE LIFE™

We inspire and enable people to improve their lives and the world around them

For more of our products visit **rodalestore.com** or call 800-848-4735

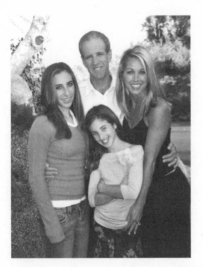

To my sweet Jeff, who always puts our family first.
And to my true joys in life, my girls, Kelly and Katie.

CONTENTS

ACKNOWLEDGMENTS

I feel so blessed to have a close-knit family and such wonderful friends. That's what life is all about—family and friends.

To my sweet mom in heaven who I miss so, so much. And to my dad for your endless support and love. I'm ever so grateful for my three awesome sisters and my great brother. We all have so much fun together. Thanks!

Without my honey bunny, Jeff, I would not have had the freedom to live this dream. Thank you, Jeff, for our happy life together as a family. You are so loving and supportive, and you always make me laugh. God bless our precious daughters, Kelly and Katie, who are growing up so fast. I love being your mom.

I want to thank Alisa Bauman for all her help with this book. You're a joy to work with. Also, thanks to Tracy Gensler, MS, RD, for her help with planning nutritious meals. A huge thank you goes to my editor, Mariska van Aalst, for believing in this project from the beginning.

Thanks to all of my friends at Lions Gate for making my videos and DVDs so successful. Thank you, Steve Beeks, Anne Parducci, and Kajsa Vikman. A special thanks to Cal Pozo, Bill Strohmeier, and Lisa Wheeler. I love you guys!

I really want to thank everyone at Waterfront Media for making the DeniseAustin.com Web site such a valuable tool for so many people who want to lose weight and feel good about themselves. It's a great feeling to know I can help people make a positive difference in their lives.

PART ONE

TUMMY TRUTHS

1 YOU CAN TONE YOUR TUMMY

**To Shed Tummy Fat for Good,
You Must Zero In on Your Unique Tummy Type**

Welcome to the Tone Your Tummy Type program! This tummy-slimming plan addresses the number one question people ask me wherever I go: "How do I flatten my tummy?" Well, throughout the pages of this book, you will discover the revolutionary answer to that question. And I'm very proud of you for taking a giant first step toward a healthier body.

It doesn't matter how stubbornly fat seems to cling to your midsection. It doesn't matter how hard or long you've tried to shrink that fat and tone that tummy. No matter how out of shape or in shape, no matter your age or your unique genetics, no matter whether you are struggling to get back in shape after having a baby or trying to halt middle-aged abdominal spread, this plan works. This plan will finally—once and for all—help you to slim down and tighten up your number one trouble spot.

A flat tummy gives you a sense of freedom. You don't have to cover up, wearing big shirts or elastic-waist pants to disguise it—you're free to wear belts, tuck in your blouse, wear cute form-fitting tops, maybe even sport a bikini again! You have more energy and confidence and less back pain or breathlessness, and you don't have any of those embarrassing rolls when you sit down. Most important, a flat tummy signals that you've minimized the very serious health risks that are associated with extra abdominal fat. When you lose belly fat, you reduce your risk of diabetes, heart disease, stroke, cancer, and many other life-threatening conditions. That power to feel healthy and strong and sexy and alive is what I want for you, and that is why I've created this plan.

Why am I so confident that the Tone Your Tummy Type program will finally enable you to successfully slim down and firm up? I know because this plan is based on many years of research—research completed at prestigious institutions across the country and even around the world. You see, over the years, medical researchers have put a lot of time and energy into finding a cure for abdominal fat gain. They've conducted thousands of studies in many different laboratory settings, looking at how various foods, supplements, exercise routines, and lifestyle habits affected abdominal fat levels in both animals and humans.

This book—for the first time—addresses the little-known fact that not all belly flab is created equal. There are five unique and distinct reasons why women gain abdominal fat. The program combines these startling study results and new thinking and assembles them into a comprehensive, effective, and realistic program that works, simply and effectively, for every body type.

When I designed this plan, I made sure to focus only on *realistic* tummy-slimming strategies. That's one of the reasons why I'm so confident this plan will work for you, no matter your history with fitness and weight gain or loss. With this plan, you will lose several inches around your middle in just 2 weeks!

I'm willing to bet that you're busy. Whether you're a stay-at-home mom, a working mom, a single-career woman, or even a retiree, you probably don't have a lot of spare time on your hands. You need something that works, works fast, and works without a lot of fuss on your part. That's what the Tone Your Tummy Type program is all about. You'll find a healthy eating plan to help you lose weight, exercises to flatten your tummy and shrink your waistline, and a comprehensive plan that really works! The recipes not only include the most effective tummy-firming ingredients but also taste delicious and are quick and simple to make. Also key, you'll find that the most picky of young eaters in your household will love them. The fitness plan includes beginner options and requires very little equipment, so you can do it at home, at your convenience, and fit it in your schedule.

If you've battled tummy fat for many years, then you've probably read and heard about numerous so-called proven ways to shrink your middle. You might even feel overwhelmed by it all. Unlike other tummy-slimming plans, the Tone Your Tummy Type program zeros in on the specific reasons why you tend to store excess fat in your abdomen. Increasing your fiber, upping your exercise time, doing more crunches, cutting back on saturated fat, quitting smoking, giving up alcohol, meditating, and much more can all work—for some people but not for others.

You see, although many women and men rank their tummy as their number one trouble spot, few women and men gain tummy fat for the same reasons. Once you discover the unique reasons why you tend to gain fat in your tummy, you can take effective action to trim down quickly, effectively, and for good.

During the next 4 weeks, you will embark on an invigorating yet very simple program—designed specifically for your tummy type—that will help you to shrink tummy fat and firm up your entire midsection. You'll trim inches from your waist but also zap that annoying back fat and those bewildering love handles (just where did they come from?). And, as a bonus, your entire body will feel firmer—your legs will have less jiggle, your buns will feel higher and tighter, and your arms will stop flapping when you wave. After you reach your weight-loss goal, you'll look leaner and longer—even more exciting, you'll feel fantastic. You'll finally be able to zip up your jeans with ease. You'll not only feel more comfortable in all of your "skinny" clothes, you may even find yourself going out and buying new outfits you never before would have considered—just to show off your amazing tummy!

Most important, however, you'll live longer and better. Shrinking abdominal fat and toning your midsection will reduce your risk of just about every disease you can think of. You'll sleep more soundly at night, feel happier, and start living the life you know you deserve. Sounds good, huh? No time to waste—let's get started so you can start feeling great today!

The Tone Your Tummy Type program is a two-phase plan. Phase 1—what I call the tummy-trimming Jump-Start Phase—lasts 2 weeks. During this phase of the plan, you can expect dramatic results. In a test group of roughly 20 people who tried the plan before it went to press, several participants lost 5, 7, or even 10 pounds during this phase. These women

I TONED MY TUMMY!

BARB HENN
TUMMY TYPE: **After Baby**
AGE: **41**
HOMETOWN: **Lisle, Illinois**
RESULTS: **Lost 15 pounds and 5 inches from her waist and tummy area in 4 weeks**
LIFE-CHANGING EXPERIENCE: **Feels stronger, both mentally and physically**

Jimmy Carter once said, "My faith demands that I do whatever I can, wherever I am, whenever I can, for as long as I can with whatever I have to try to make a difference."

My weight—particularly, my tummy—had gotten out of control, and it was time for me to follow former President Carter's motto and do whatever I could to make a difference.

I also recently had a bout with cancer, and I wanted to make sure my body would be prepared to fight in case disease should strike again. Denise Austin's Tone Your Tummy Type program gave me the tools and motivation I needed to get started.

I think the bulk of my tummy problems came from my three C-sections. I had three big babies—11 pounds, 12 ounces; 11 pounds, 7 ounces; and 8 pounds, 8 ounces (my peanut). The stretching from the pregnancies, combined with the injury from the C-sections, made it very difficult for me to regain a flat tummy.

But the real start of my weight battle began long before I became pregnant, when I got married and moved away from my family to attend college with my spouse. It was a bad relationship that went on for 17 years. Without my family to lean on, I used food for support. I was raised in a family where food was always a key player in family gatherings, so it was the first thing I turned to for comfort. Luckily, I turned my life around—I got divorced and lost 100 pounds.

But old habits die hard. . . .

During my second marriage, I started to slip back into my previous bad eating habits; as in many families, there were lots of outings that centered on food. Then, after my third pregnancy, I went back to work full-time. The combination of the food outings and the more sedentary lifestyle led me to gain back 60 pounds of what I had lost. Being fat made me feel miserable, especially when I had to shop for clothes.

shrunk many inches off their waistlines (and their thighs and hips) in just 2 weeks. All the while, they raved about their increased energy levels. Almost immediately, they stopped having cravings. And they stuck with the meal plan effortlessly—some even said the plans called for too much food!

So needless to say, I had to do something. The Tone Your Tummy Type program came along at the perfect time. My motivation for starting the program was certainly not to win beauty contests but to be able to buy clothes easily and to be healthy for myself and my children.

The Tone Your Tummy Type program has definitely given me the jump-start I needed to shrink my tummy. First, I now realize how much I really was eating in the past—my portion sizes were way too big! I guess when I was young and really active, it didn't matter. But now that I'm older, I don't have a choice. In order to keep my weight and my tummy under control, I have to eat less. Period. Denise's Tone Your Tummy Type program has made me constantly conscious of how much I eat at home, at restaurants, and at family gatherings. I am forever going to eat half of what I used to consume.

In addition, the Tone Your Tummy Type program has taught me to appreciate new foods. I have changed over to soy butter products and olive oil for cooking, and I have a new love of yogurt, particularly the Stonyfield brand. I add yogurt to the shakes and smoothies I make for myself and my children.

I also truly enjoy the recipes in the plan. I particularly love the breakfasts out! I prefer to eat out at breakfast time. I find it satisfying and less expensive, and, by eating in the morning, I feel like I'm working off more calories throughout the day.

My favorite recipes include the Pinto Bean Bowl and the Bean Dip. They are fantastic!

The exercises in the Tone Your Tummy Type program are both effective and easy to do. I know that with my body type and metabolism, I have to move to lose weight, so an exercise program that fits well into my lifestyle and schedule is important.

Overall, the fabulous results I've seen so far on this program have made me feel more successful as a person. People have already noticed my weight loss. The other day, when I was heading out to exercise, my husband asked how much weight I have lost. When I told him, he said it looked like much more than that—so obviously, the pounds are coming off in all the right places! Seeing the weight come off and knowing I will lose more in the future feels wonderful. I am stronger, mentally and physically.

Thanks, Denise!

Once you've completed phase 1, you'll move on to phase 2—what I call the tummy-tightening Keep-On-Losing Phase. You'll be able to eat even more food and get into a rhythm with your exercise that will help your body continue to shed up to 2 pounds a week. You'll need only 2 weeks to see results and 4 weeks to complete the Tone Your Tummy Type program. If you'd like to keep losing, I'll give you tips on how to tweak and modify the plan so you can stay on it and continue shedding pounds and inches. Once you've reached your goal, I'll help you maintain your amazing body, for good.

MY TUMMY TYPE—AND YOURS

Okay, I'll admit it: For most of my life, I've been a bit lucky when it comes to my tummy. Throughout the years, I've tended to gain weight in my thighs but not in my tummy. Consequently, during much of my career, I've had firm abs and have even been known to lift up my shirt and dare television hosts and others to "feel my tummy"!

Even after the births of my daughters during my thirties, I was able to quickly firm up my abs. In fact, I was filming videos and my television show just 6 weeks after giving birth to each of my baby girls! My tummy, of course, wasn't rock hard just 6 weeks postpartum. It was still a little poochy and thick around the middle, but flat enough that the softness didn't show up on TV. By about 6 months after giving birth to my first and 9 months after giving birth to my second daughter, my tummy had bounced back to its former flat and firm self.

But then, in my midforties, things began to change. It seemed as if little culinary indiscretions—the small bites of macaroni and cheese I sneaked off my daughters' plates or the sweets I allowed myself in the afternoon—seemed to settle below my belly button. If I slacked off on my abdominal exercise, my tummy seemed to instantly become poochy and soft.

I knew what could happen if I allowed this trend to continue. I'd seen it firsthand. The women in my family have a tendency toward gaining tummy fat, especially after menopause. I wasn't about to let this happen. As someone whose business it is to know all about fitness, I am well aware of the dangers of abdominal fat and the health risks associated with allowing it to accumulate. At the same time, I didn't want to give up eating the foods I loved. I didn't want to exercise even harder and longer than I already was. It just didn't seem possible. It didn't seem fair. "There must be a better way," I thought.

To find a better way, I began talking to the country's top doctors and experts, researching the medical literature, and experimenting with new and unique fitness routines that target the tummy in innovative ways.

I know that there is just one way to lose weight: Eat less and exercise more. This tried-and-true formula has kept me and many of my fans fit for more than 25 years. Yet, I learned that while exercise and healthful eating certainly form the foundation of every good tummy-trimming plan, this foundation should be built slightly differently depending on the source of the problem.

I learned that women tend to fall into five different tummy types, all with differing needs. These five different types gain abdominal fat for different reasons and, therefore, need different plans to lose that fat and firm up the midsection. Men, on the other hand, face different challenges; I created a program to help guys tackle their guts, too.

In the coming pages you'll learn more about the tummy types and will take a quiz that will help you to determine your type. With your quiz results, you'll be able to turn to your specific tummy type chapter and find your unique recipe for slimming down and firming up—for good.

When I determined my personal tummy type, I found out that I could keep it under control pretty simply. Although I am not menopausal yet, I'm coming up on my 50th birthday. I haven't noticed any perimenopausal symptoms (no hot flashes or night sweats!), but I do see my body starting to change. In years past, I've tended to gain weight in my thighs—and not my tummy. Now that I'm approaching menopause, however, my tummy type has begun to shift. For that reason, I've used the Peri/Postmenopause Tummy Type program. My personal recipe involves doing 3 to 5 minutes of abdominal exercises a day, reining in salty processed foods that were bloating my tummy, and constantly working on my posture. Once I focused on a few additional key eating, exercise, and lifestyle strategies proven to work for my tummy type, I found I could much more effortlessly keep my tummy flat below the navel and firm all over. Just a few tweaks was all it took!

ONE CORE PLAN

No matter your tummy type, you'll enjoy a delicious eating plan and an energizing exercise plan. In Parts 3 and 4 of this book, you will find a fitness and eating plan that helps all tummy types whittle away belly fat and firm up abdominal flab. I've worked hard to ensure that this plan includes the very best of the latest and most effective routines for trimming your midriff and slimming your waistline.

My Core Moves plan focuses on three essential but often underplayed types of exercise to help you burn fat and trim tummy flab. I've divided the plan into two phases, each of which lasts 2 weeks. For each phase of the plan, you'll find two exercise routines that effectively combine all of the fitness elements you need to shrink your waistline and flatten your tummy. The combination movements in these routines have been proven to burn fat *three times faster* than traditional exercise programs!

Specifically, the plan includes cardio to burn the fat that's hiding that beautiful waistline of yours. It includes strength training to build lean, sexy muscle that helps boost your metabolism. Finally, it includes tummy-sculpting movements to firm up flab. Think of these routines as multitasking routines, because the innovative movements allow you to accomplish many of those important fitness goals at once. For example, some of the strength-training moves will simultaneously get your heart rate up to burn fat. Some of the cardio moves will also tone your abs.

Exercise is only part of the picture. My Core Diet includes an eating plan created to speed weight loss while it reduces inflammation in your body. Emerging research has linked inflammation throughout the body with abdominal fat (see "What Is Inflammation?"). Scientists are starting to see that if you reduce the inflammation, you shed the belly fat—especially that stubborn abdominal fat that seems to cling to your body no matter how many crunches you complete!

This inflammation-reducing diet showcases natural foods high in fiber, omega-3 fatty acids, and phytonutrients from fruits and vegetables. It minimizes overly refined carbohydrates, added sugar, saturated fats, and trans fats, all of which increase inflammation and contribute to abdominal fat.

WHAT IS INFLAMMATION?

Inflammation can be a good thing. It's a process in which the body's white blood cells and chemicals can protect us from infection and foreign substances such as bacteria and viruses. When inflammation occurs, chemicals from the body's white blood cells are released into the blood or affected tissues. This release increases the blood flow to an area of injury or infection, and it may result in redness or a feeling of warmth. Some of the chemicals cause a leak of fluid into the tissues, resulting in swelling.

When it comes to inflammation, some is good but more is not better. Too much inflammation affects every part of your body negatively. Researchers now believe that too much inflammation may trigger heart disease, some cancers, and even joint pain. It even seems to disrupt the metabolism, as several studies have found a link between abdominal fat and markers of chronic inflammation. You'll learn more about this important connection in Chapter 2.

To ensure that you see success quickly, I've organized the meal plan as well into two phases that span 2 weeks each. On the phase 1 meal plan, you will consume 1,300 daily calories, a calorie level that will jump-start your weight loss, leading to rapid initial results, without leaving you feeling deprived or hungry. In phase 2, you'll get to eat even more food, for a combined total of 1,500 calories a day. During this phase, you'll continue to lose weight at a fast but sustainable pace that will ensure your results last for the long term. You'll learn more about this tasty and simple yet powerful eating plan in Chapter 10.

What I find very exciting about this plan is that while the "core" program works for everyone, your results will be enhanced and multiplied just by taking your own tummy type into account. Once you discover your unique tummy type in Chapter 3, you will use the tips in Chapters 4 through 9 to customize the Tone Your Tummy Type program to your specific tummy needs. For example, some types will add a little more exercise than prescribed in the core program. Other types will focus on important lifestyle changes in addition to the core plan. Still other types will slightly modify the eating plan.

OF TUMMY TRUTHS AND TUMMY MYTHS

When I talk to the visitors of my Web site (DeniseAustin.com) or read letters from viewers of my TV shows, I can see that trimming tummy fat can seem pretty confusing. Marketers know that you want to slim down your midsection, so many supplements, diets, lifestyle tips, pieces of exercise equipment, and fitness spas claim to help you do just that. But the conflicts between all the different claims are enough to drive you crazy! That's why I wrote this book—to sort through the noise and just tell you what *works*.

In fact, before we delve any deeper into the specifics of the Tone Your Tummy Type plan, let's look at some of the confusing messages you may have heard before—and why you may have been saddled with a larger belly than you wanted up until now. Once you know the truth, you'll be better equipped to confidently embark on the Tone Your Tummy Type program and lose tummy fat for good.

MYTH: There's only one way to shrink your tummy.

FACT: There are many effective ways to burn tummy fat. The best strategy for you will zero in on the unique reasons why you gain fat in your tummy to begin with. A woman, for example, who was slender most of her life only to start gaining fat at menopause needs a very different plan than a younger woman who has battled tummy fat as far back as she can remember. Whereas hormones are causing the first woman to gain tummy fat, genetics may be to blame for the latter woman's struggle. As a result, some women experience lasting visible benefits from relaxation therapies, whereas other women find stress reduction does nothing to whittle away their tummy fat.

To trim your middle, you must understand why the fat is there in the first place. No matter your tummy type, you must, of course, feed your body well and make sure you move enough, but some types need to exercise less than others, and some types need to follow a slightly less strict diet than others. You'll find out how to put together the right tummy-slimming essentials for you throughout the pages of this book!

MYTH: There's only one type of tummy fat: the type that makes it impossible to zip up your jeans.

FACT: Abdominal fat comes in many varieties. The pinchable fat just below the skin is called subcutaneous fat. This is the fat you can see, touch, and jiggle. The deeper fat packed in and around the GI system is called visceral fat. This hard fat accumulates so deeply in the abdomen that you might not even notice its presence. That's right—some people with flat tummies have abnormally high amounts of visceral fat. Fat can also accumulate in the liver and in the omentum, an organ that hangs beneath your stomach. Of all the types of abdominal fat, visceral fat is the most dangerous to your health. A study conducted at the Cooper Clinic in Dallas determined that the more visceral fat you have, the higher your risk of death during the following 3 years.

MYTH: Crunches are the best way to shrink your tummy.

FACT: Although crunches and other abdominal exercises will strengthen and sculpt muscle in your tummy, they won't shrink the fat that hides that beautiful muscle. To show off that beautiful tummy you've done so many crunches to create, you need a comprehensive plan that includes diet, cardio, and weight training to boost metabolism and burn fat.

MYTH: You must eat less to shrink your tummy, even if that means feeling hungry all day long and going to bed dreaming of food.

FACT: When you crash-diet to lose weight, you set yourself up for failure. Roughly 7 of every 10 pounds of weight lost through crash dieting comes from muscle and not from fat tissue! Because muscle tissue is metabolically active—with each pound burning between 35 and 50 calories a day—your success lies in gaining muscle tissue, not in losing it! Losing muscle tissue slows your metabolism, which creates the following vicious cycle: A slower metabolism means you must eat less and less food to maintain your weight loss. This constant food restriction leaves you feeling hungry and deprived, which eventually causes you to overeat and gain weight.

Don't get me wrong. To lose weight, you must eat less. That said, you do not need to restrict calories to the point of near starvation! As I mentioned, the Core Diet plan includes two phases, with the first phase consisting of 1,300 calories a day, a calorie level determined by a nutritionist to be ideal for fast, lasting results. This calorie amount is low enough to trigger weight loss, but high enough to do so without leaving you hungry, tired, and deprived. After 2 weeks, you'll step up your calorie intake to 1,500 daily calories, enough to leave you satisfied, but still low enough to allow you to continue losing weight.

The Tone Your Tummy Type program combines this two-phase eating plan with cardio and weight training to ensure that the weight you lose comes from fat—and not from muscle. Research shows that combining dieting with cardio slows muscle tissue loss, but that only resistance training (as prescribed in this program) prevents muscle loss altogether.

Another reason to combine diet with exercise: Research from Japan shows that dieting tends to burn off just one type of tummy fat—the dangerous visceral fat (learn more about different types of abdominal fat in Chapter 2). Exercise, on the other hand, tends to target the jiggly, more noticeable subcutaneous fat stored just beneath your skin. The combination of the right diet and and the right exercises will truly tame tummy fat for good.

MYTH: Cardio does nothing to shrink your tummy.

FACT: Cardio will help you to burn excess calories, maximizing your success. It also may help you to stick with the Core Diet plan, as many aerobically fit exercisers lose their taste for processed and sugary foods and develop a taste for fruits, vegetables, and other wholesome, high-fiber foods once they start doing regular cardio. Finally, regular cardio will also help you to keep off your tummy fat once you lose it. The National Weight Control Registry has tracked the weight-loss methods of thousands of women and men who have lost at least 30 pounds and kept it off for a year or longer. Results from the registry show that successful dieters consistently use cardio as a way to maintain their weight loss.

MYTH: To shrink your tummy, you don't need to lift weights.

FACT: You'd be missing out on a great tummy-shrinking secret if you don't use weights. A study of 30 obese women determined that participants who combined cardio with weight training lost three times as much subcutaneous (beneath the skin) abdominal fat and 13 percent more visceral abdominal fat (packed around the internal organs) as the women who only did cardio.

MYTH: To shed abdominal fat fast, you should do as much exercise as possible.

FACT: You can actually overdo it when it comes to exercise. Too much exercise is a physical stressor that triggers your adrenal glands to release the stress hormone cortisol (especially in women), one of the very hormones responsible for the storage of tummy fat! Too much exercise can also reduce testosterone levels, a side effect that's desirable for some tummy types but not for most. This muscle-building hormone (which, despite popular belief, is present in both sexes in differing amounts) is involved in fat burning. In order not to overdo it too quickly, the Core Moves plan starts slow—with just 10 to 20 minutes of exercise 5 days a week during phase 1. In phase 2, you'll kick it up a notch—but not push yourself beyond your comfort zone. The bottom line: You must exercise more efficiently and smarter—but do not overdo it!

MYTH: Breastfeeding helps all new moms lose their tummy fat.

FACT: It's true that breastfeeding burns roughly 500 calories a day, the equivalent of walking or running 5 miles. So, for many women, breastfeeding does enable weight loss. That said, for other women it does not. In these women, breastfeeding seems to signal the body to hold tightly to its fat stores, consequently slowing the metabolism. The good news is that many women find that once they stop nursing and continue their weight-loss efforts, the fat comes right off. (And one of the tummy type programs is here to help!)

MYTH: You have a big belly because you eat too much.

FACT: Although overeating can certainly lead to tummy fat—especially if you are prone to gaining fat in the abdomen—it's not the only cause of abdominal fat gain. You may gain fat in your abdomen for any number of reasons, including your personal genetics and your lifestyle (stress, smoking, and alcohol consumption all lead to tummy fat).

MYTH: The only thing you need to shrink your tummy is the ab machine you saw advertised on TV.

FACT: I'm a big believer in exercise equipment if it motivates or enables you to exercise when you otherwise would not be able to (for example, by eliminating neck discomfort of typical abdominal exercises). That said, no piece of equipment to date works like magic to shrink your middle. Ab machines simply make exercising your abdomen easier or more effective by promoting proper form. If a layer of fat covers your abdominal muscles, sculpting those muscles with a machine will do only one thing: make that layer of fat more noticeable! To shrink your middle, you need to work on sculpting your abs, but you also must burn off the fat that hides those beautiful muscles. To do that you need a sensible diet and moderate cardio and strength training. So use a machine if you like, but don't use it as the one and only ingredient in your tummy-slimming plan.

MYTH: Fat-burning supplements don't ever work.

FACT: Although old-school fat-burning supplements like ephedra were bad for your health and eventually taken off the market, some other supplements do show some promise when it comes to trimming tummy fat.

I TONED MY TUMMY!

KARLA SCHUHOW
TUMMY TYPE: **Apple**
AGE: **43**
HOMETOWN: **Bellingham, Washington**
RESULTS: **Lost 11 pounds and 6½ inches off her waist in 4 weeks**
LIFE-CHANGING EXPERIENCE: **Has tremendous energy and clearer skin**

Over the years, as my stomach grew, my self-esteem shrunk. Although I never had a six-pack, I never had a bulge either, until recently. I became constantly aware of and overwhelmed by my tummy. I just didn't feel as if I looked good in anything. Plus, my cholesterol level was rising. It was time for me to fight back. Denise Austin's Tone Your Tummy Type program immediately spoke to me.

The main thing that drew me to the program was the balanced meal plan. The food is flavorful and "normal," and the recipes are easy to follow and to work into my day. The dinners incorporate a variety of colors and textures, and my whole family loves them!

My first impression of the program was right on; it was exactly what I needed to get on track toward a positive change. On Day 4, I already noticed a decrease in my appetite. Then, after only 1 week on the Tone Your Tummy Type program, I had a ton more energy, and I could see my body changing shape.

The exercises quickly became a part of my routine, and I instantly felt more flexible. I don't have much natural flexibility, but I now have a larger range of motion in my neck, and my back feels a lot stronger.

The Tone Your Tummy Type program has also made me conscious of what and how much I

I recommend fish oil for all tummy types. Various studies done on rats and on humans show that fish oil seems to inhibit abdominal fat. In one of these studies, participants who took 6 grams of fish oil daily and exercised for 3 months reduced abdominal fat by 5 percent. Participants who only exercised but did not take fish oil or only took fish oil but did not exercise lost no abdominal fat.

Fish oil may help you shed fat by increasing the number of fat-burning enzymes in your body. It may also help to lower abdominal fat through its anti-inflammatory properties. A key anti-inflammatory fat in humans is derived from a fatty acid found in fish oil.

I personally take 1,200 milligrams of odorless omega-3 fatty acids a day. Although

was eating. Before I started the program, I ate way too many calories. I now use my food scale and measuring cups every day. I used to crave junk food, but now I reach for fresh fruit and veggies for a snack—and I don't mind! I love eating healthful food, and I actually look forward to salads. (I never knew I liked couscous!)

I also keep water bottles at my desk at work, and I make sure I always have one in the car. I finish at least one bottle of water before I get to work. Then, for a work snack, I eat the Tone Your Tummy Type On-the-Go Muffins. They're so easy to make and really stick with me. I bake them on Sunday evening, put them into sandwich bags, throw them into the freezer, and grab one each morning. I have one at about 10:00 a.m., and then I'm full until lunch!

Physically, I feel awesome on this program—so energetic! My tummy has been a little sore from the routines, but it's a good sore. At one point on the plan, everyone in my family was sick, but I staved it off. I think the exercise and healthy food helped keep me well!

I have definitely gotten the results I had hoped to get in 4 weeks. I lost 11 pounds this month and 6½ inches off my waist. People have started to ask me if I'm losing weight. . . .

Aside from my weight and health, my complexion has been so clear since I started the Tone Your Tummy Type program. My skin is soft and smooth, and I've actually gotten just as many compliments on my complexion as I have on my weight loss—I'm glowing!

I am so thrilled that I decided to try Denise's Tone Your Tummy Type program. It's a well-balanced plan with wholesome food and exercises that are easy to follow and incorporate into my day. It gave me the start I needed for a total lifestyle change. I feel so encouraged by my results, and I'm eager to continue. I plan to use the Tone Your Tummy Type program to reach my ultimate weight-loss goal (34 pounds). Thus far, it has been such a pleasure! Thanks, Denise!

many lab tests show that most commercial fish oil supplements contain no or far less mercury and other contaminants as regular fish, I recommend you look for a "purified" supplement. And, as I recommend for all supplements, check with your doctor before taking fish oil, especially if you are breastfeeding or taking blood-thinning medication.

MYTH: You can never shrink your tummy (because you think you're too fat or too out of shape).

FACT: Everyone has what it takes to shrink their middle! Although the quest for a trim waistline may be more challenging for some people than others, many scientific studies show that the right exercise, eating, and lifestyle changes work very effectively at trimming tummy fat. You can do it, and you have what it takes!

I'm a firm believer that no one is too large or too out of shape to get back in shape! To make a new habit like exercise last, take small baby steps, starting with a duration and intensity that you can handle and building from there. I designed the phase 1 routines in this book for beginners, but if the exercises feel too challenging for you, go easy on yourself, cutting out certain exercises or doing fewer reps. Listen to your body, pushing yourself to your edge—but not beyond it.

MYTH: You're a veteran yo-yo dieter. That's why you have tummy fat.

FACT: Yo-yo dieting may have slowed your metabolism over the years—which means you'll gain weight more easily and have to work harder to lose it—but it probably did not change your body shape or fat distribution. A number of factors influence whether you store fat in your middle—and you'll learn about all of them throughout the pages of this book—but weight cycling is not one of them.

MYTH: Smoking helps burn calories. You'll get even fatter if you quit.

FACT: Although many smokers do find that their metabolism slows down when they quit—sometimes triggering weight gain—they also find that smoking cessation changes their body shape for the better. Research published in the journal *Obesity Research* shows that cigarette smoking leads to increased levels of abdominal fat. This study evaluated the height, weight, waist circumference, hip circumference, and smoking history of 21,828 British men and women. The study found that current smokers had higher waist-to-hip ratios and waist circumferences than nonsmokers or recovering smokers. Although the current smokers tended to weigh less on the scale than nonsmokers, they tended to pack all of their excess body fat into one place—their abdomens.

MYTH: Cholesterol levels are the only things that affect heart health.

FACT: High cholesterol levels identify less than half of people who are at risk of having a heart attack, which is why you may know of people who received a normal cholesterol reading one day and suffered a heart attack the next.

Although cholesterol may cause some heart attacks, inflammation probably causes many more. Inflammation is the process that causes redness and swelling around an injury. When the inflammatory process becomes chronic—as it does when you carry excess fat around the middle—it leads to heart disease, even if your cholesterol numbers are normal. People with abdominal fat tend to have higher levels of C-reactive protein (CRP), a key marker of inflammation and heart disease risk. If you have not done so already, consider asking your doctor to test your CRP levels. Anything higher than 10 milligrams per liter (mg/l) is considered elevated, an indication that too much inflammation is taking place in your body. The results may surprise you—and solidify your motivation to stick to your own Tone Your Tummy Type plan.

So now you know the truth about what it takes to shrink tummy fat. You're about to embark on an exciting program. It will without a doubt change the shape of your body for the better. I know you are already motivated—raring to go. Otherwise you wouldn't be holding this book in your hands. But I want you to get even more motivated. The more motivated you are to change on Day 1, the more motivation you'll have to carry you through the tough times. So turn to Chapter 2 to find out some very compelling reasons to shed tummy fat—reasons that, until now, you may not have ever read about.

2 TAMING TUMMY TROUBLE

Motivating reasons to change for the better

You might think of belly fat in terms of its appearance. It's the stuff that hangs off your middle, making you feel too self-conscious to buy new clothes or wear a bikini or, if you're a man, go shirtless. But the lumpy belly that can be an annoyance in the dressing room might someday also prompt a trip to the emergency room!

Although appearance alone can certainly motivate you to change your diet, start an exercise program, and incorporate other lifestyle changes needed to shrink tummy fat and firm tummy flab, in this chapter I'd like to talk to you about another motivating reason to shrink your middle—your health. Consider:

* Research of more than 27,000 people that was published in the prestigious medical journal *The Lancet* determined that your waist measurement—and not your overall level of body fat or your weight—is the best predictor of whether you will develop heart disease.

* A report from Kaiser Permanente this year concluded that people with

the most abdominal fat were nearly 2½ times more likely to develop dementia as people with the least abdominal fat.

* Various studies have linked high amounts of abdominal fat with an increased risk of gallstones, breast cancer, and premature death.

* According to a study published in *Obesity Research,* a man with 2.2 pounds of abdominal fat has double the risk of death, compared with a man with 1.1 pounds of fat.

How does abdominal fat negatively affect so many parts of the body? Scientists lump abdominal fat in the same category as the heart, liver, and other *organs.* That's right, abdominal fat is an organ, complete with endocrine cells that secrete hormones (such as leptin) and inflammation-producing cytokines. It also has its own blood supply. The substances produced in your abdominal fat send messages to many bodily organs, triggering a cascade of ill effects, including inflammation. As you'll soon learn, too much inflammation can erode the health of your entire body, including the health of your heart and your metabolism.

By embarking on the Tone Your Tummy Type program, you're about to halt the tummy fat–inflammation cycle. I'm excited to tell you that research has shown time and time again that reducing abdominal fat—even by just a little bit—goes a long way toward improving your overall health.

It's my hope that the information you find in this chapter will help to further fuel your motivation to embark on and stick with the Tone Your Tummy Type program. It's one thing to lose weight to fit into your favorite pair of jeans. It's quite another to do so to save your life! Once you understand the science behind how the body stores and uses tummy fat, you'll have the foundation you need to understand the importance of all of the elements of the Tone Your Tummy Type program.

THE SKINNY ON BELLY FAT

Many people think there are only two types of fat—the fat stored in your thighs and hips (creating a "pear" shape) and the fat stored in your tummy (creating an "apple" shape). In reality, the body contains many different types of fat, and not all of these types of fat affect your health equally.

Just in the tummy alone, there are four sources of fat.

Subcutaneous: This pinchable fat lies just beneath the skin. It's the fat you can see when someone's tummy sways and jiggles. This type of fat does not tend to affect health as adversely as other types of abdominal fat.

I TONED MY TUMMY!

APRIL BROWN
TUMMY TYPE: **Stressed Slender**
AGE: **33**
HOMETOWN: **West Linn, Oregon**
RESULTS: **9 pounds and 11 total inches lost in 4 weeks**
LIFE-CHANGING EXPERIENCE: **Fits back into her size 8 jeans again and is a knockout in a bikini**

Before Denise's program, I had the classic stress tummy. With four young children, I get little time for myself. Plus, my husband works days, Monday through Friday, and I work nights and weekends part-time to make ends meet. Because of my busy schedule, I got into an unhealthy pattern of being tired, eating poorly, feeling tired from the bad food, and then not exercising because I was too tired. I have a genetic tendency to gain weight in my stomach and upper thighs, so my bad habits manifested themselves as fat in those areas.

I have been a relatively thin person throughout my life (too thin in my twenties), so the extra 10 pounds I was carrying in my tummy and thighs weighed heavily on my mind. I have a long torso, so one-piece bathing suits never fit me correctly; instead, I was forced to wear a bikini with shorts over it to hold in my belly and thighs. I used to be *constantly* embarrassed about my stomach.

I tried vegetarian diets to lose the weight, but I just didn't feel good on them. I am a huge Denise Austin fan (my mom first introduced me to Denise in the 1990s), so when I heard about the Tone Your Tummy Type program, I immediately wanted to take on the challenge.

I had two motivations for losing my tummy. First, I was tired of being ashamed of my appearance—I simply wanted to look better. Second, I did it for my health. I was eating a lot of snacks with my kids when they came home from school; I often ate even more of the snacks than they did! I was sick and tired of feeling bad physically. It was definitely time for me to take charge of my exercise and eating habits.

Visceral: This deep fat packed around the internal organs is not as noticeable as subcutaneous fat. In fact, many relatively slender people have dangerous amounts of visceral fat—and don't know it! Visceral fat surrounds your liver. Due to its location, it more easily breaks down and releases fatty acids into the bloodstream—where they can clog your arteries and cause other havoc—than subcutaneous fat. In fact, research shows that this fat breaks down and is resynthesized four to five times faster than fat in other parts of the body and abdomen.

Denise's program has worked very well to help me lose my tummy fat. The recipes are awesome, and they fill me up. I have learned to enjoy new foods—I never thought I would like papaya, mango, or kiwifruit, but they are delicious! I was also a little wary of the Cabbage Apple Salad at first, but it's one of my favorite recipes now. I drink flavored seltzer water as a treat—a great alternative to soda, and even my kids enjoy it.

I love being able to eat four times a day on this program. I also like the specificity of the recipes—they have helped me learn portion control, a skill I will use forever. I now weigh and measure everything I eat.

In addition, the program has taught me the power of protein—my energy level skyrocketed in the first 2 days on the plan, which I attribute to the high protein content. I have also learned the importance of toning. Before I started the program, I only weight trained once a week. With the regular toning exercises in the Tone Your Tummy Type program, I noticed a significant difference in my body after only 2 weeks. First, my energy came back, and then the fat just started melting away. I lost 8 inches off my body in the first week alone!

Two weeks into Denise Austin's Tone Your Tummy Type program, I actually found sugar sickening. One day my husband brought me what used to be my favorite treat—a nonfat no-whip mocha—and it was *so sweet*. I did not enjoy it at all, and I felt really sick after I finished it. I think I'll get the plain lattes and skip all of that sugar from now on!

My desire for *all* junk foods has faded as well. I now feel as if I can control my junk food cravings; the cravings no longer control me! My family joined me on the program, and since adding more protein and making the other healthful changes, we're all in better moods. We're healthier and less stressed, thanks to the Tone Your Tummy Type program!

When I started Denise's program, my goal was to look fabulous in a bikini this summer. My husband said I looked great before, but I wanted to be a *knockout* for him and myself. I totally succeeded! I will definitely continue with the program in the future to maintain this healthier, more attractive, and happier me.

Liver fat: Your liver stores fat and sugar for later use. As a result, when you are overweight, the cells inside your liver can start to fill up with fat, creating a "fatty liver." If your fatty liver is caused by obesity—and not by alcoholism—it usually does not lead to liver disease and usually can be reversed with weight loss. If enough fat accumulates in the liver, however, liver disease can occur.

Omentum fat: Few people have heard of the omentum, an organ that hangs beneath your stomach. It holds on to and stores the excess fat calories from your food. When your body stores calories in this fatty pouch, it has easy access to it. The more easily fat is mobilized, the more easily it can enter your bloodstream and end up in places where it should not, such as inside other bodily organs.

Exactly why tummy fat leads to health problems isn't entirely clear, and many researchers around the world are spending a lot of time trying to unravel this mystery. One popular theory holds that tummy fat—especially visceral fat—tends to drain into the liver. The liver breaks down these fats, which then leave the liver and enter the bloodstream in the form of triglycerides (a type of blood fat).

Your body tries to regulate the amount of fat in your bloodstream, so when your liver releases a load of triglycerides into the blood, your muscle cells and other organs attempt to soak up this fat, much like a sponge soaking up excess water. Yet, when triglycerides gum up your muscles, your muscles have a tougher time absorbing and burning sugar for energy. As a result, insulin—the chief hormone responsible for signaling your muscles to take up and burn sugar—loses its effectiveness, creating a condition known as insulin resistance. Consequently, blood sugar levels begin to rise. To drive these sugar levels down to normal levels, your pancreas secretes abnormally high amounts of insulin. For a while, these higher-than-usual amounts of insulin effectively work to shuttle sugar into cells. Over time, however, the pancreas begins to wear out, causing type 2 diabetes.

Insulin resistance is thought to cause:

1. Levels of the good HDL cholesterol to plummet
2. Increased sodium absorption in the gut, which expands your blood volume and drives up blood pressure

3. Hunger and fat storage (which leads to overeating and the creation of more tummy fat—which, in turn, furthers this vicious cycle)

In short, abdominal fat—especially visceral fat—drains away your health. It increases your risk for heart disease, diabetes, stroke, and cancer. Because of its location, it also tends to cause back pain, breathing problems, and persistent cough.

THE INFLAMMATION CYCLE

I mentioned earlier that tummy fat tends to trigger a cascade of ill health effects, including raising the level of inflammation in your body. But why exactly is inflammation bad for you?

As I mentioned in Chapter 1, inflammation is your body's first defense against disease. For example, when a virus gets into your nasal passageways, your body responds by inflaming those passageways to prevent the virus from traveling further into your body. Although this inflammation gives you the dreaded stuffy nose, it prevents you from suffering a worse fate: a chest infection.

The same type of response takes place inside your blood vessels and joints when you eat an inflammation-producing diet. Although the right amount of inflammation at the right times allows the immune system to repair damaged joints and vessels, too much inflammation on a chronic basis does the opposite—it makes you sick. A number of chemicals and messengers are involved in the inflammatory process, and, among other things, elevated levels of these chemicals make the hormones insulin and leptin work less effectively.

I've already told you what happens when insulin does not work effectively. Let's take a moment to talk about the hormone leptin.

Leptin is a hormone that regulates appetite, metabolism, and body weight. Your fat cells secrete leptin. When levels of this hormone are high, they signal the various glands in your body to turn up metabolism and turn down appetite. When you eat an inflammation-producing diet, however, something goes awry, and the brain and glands do not respond normally to fluctuations in leptin levels. So even as body fat levels go up, appetite remains the same or even increases—contributing to fat gain!

The inflammation cycle tends to perpetuate itself because abdominal fat itself secretes certain inflammation-producing immune cells called cytokines. As a result, a little abdominal fat tends to lead to a lot of abdominal fat because of the vicious inflammation cycle it creates inside the body.

HOW TO HALT THE CYCLE

Anyone who knows me knows that I'm a positive person. So, although I wanted you to understand exactly what is at stake, it's time to end this dose of bad news. I'm here to say that you can actually lose inches in your waistline! You can shrink your middle! Research done at Duke University in Durham, North Carolina, found that couch potatoes who started exercising either on a treadmill or stationary bike tended to quickly lose their visceral fat (the deep abdominal fat packed around the internal organs). The participants who did the most exercise shed both visceral and subcutaneous fat. Their peers who did not exercise, however, got fatter.

You need to lose only a small amount of abdominal fat to boost your health in a big way. Just a 5 to 10 percent reduction in tummy fat can substantially reduce your risk of diabetes and heart disease, finds research done at Laval University in Quebec.

So you can do it, and the Tone Your Tummy Type program will show you how! Throughout the pages of this book, you will find many effective strategies for trimming tummy fat and toning tummy flab—and you will learn exactly which strategies are most important to your tummy type (which you'll discover in Chapter 3). For instance, here are a few of the tummy-slimming all-stars that will be featured in Tone Your Tummy Type chapters to follow.

Reduce negative stress. Tummy fat is more sensitive to the stress hormone cortisol than other types of fat in your body. The more you experience negative stress, the more cortisol your tummy fat cells are exposed to. You can be exposed to cortisol in two ways.

1. You may have a lot of stress in your life. Perhaps you are selling a house, parenting a colicky infant, or experiencing difficulties at work or in your relationships.
2. You may react to certain stressors differently than other people would, secreting more coristol, say, when you get caught in traffic than would someone who is more laid-back.

Although reducing the amount of daily stress would help anyone, this tactic helps some tummy types more than others.

Get more sleep. Chronic sleep deprivation affects leptin, the appetite-control hormone I mentioned earlier. Produced by fat cells, leptin levels tell the brain when the body does or does not need more food. During sleep, leptin levels normally rise. Getting too few hours of sleep, however, causes other hormones to rise, which, in turn, drive down leptin levels, making you feel hungry. Although we could probably all benefit from more sleep, some tummy types benefit more than others.

Tailor your exercise plan. No matter your tummy type, you need exercise to slim down and firm up your midsection. Exercise helps to increase your metabolism (so you burn more calories), reduce appetite, and enable your body to burn fat more easily. It also keeps excess amounts of tummy fat from hindering your health. Case in point: Sumo wrestlers who may look fat and unhealthy and who eat huge amounts of food actually exercise for hours every day. Their abdominal fat is predominantly stored just below the skin, rather than deep in the abdominal cavity. Research shows that, despite their big tummies, sumo wrestlers are actually at a very low risk for heart disease.

The Tone Your Tummy Type program contains a core exercise plan for all types, but you'll learn how to modify that program when you read about your specific tummy type in Chapters 4 through 9.

Fine-tune your diet. All tummy types need to follow the inflammation-reducing eating plan laid out in Chapters 10, 12, and 13. That said, some types may need to follow this plan more strictly than others. You'll learn about additional superfoods that may speed up your success when you read about your specific tummy type in Chapters 4 through 9.

Consider fish oil supplements. In Chapter 1, I mentioned fish oil supplements. Of all of the available supplements, I feel they hold the most success in helping you trim tummy fat. I recommend fish oil for all types (possibly with the exception of women who are lactating and people who are taking blood-thinning medications).

Please stop smoking. Smoking tends to cause your body to store fat in your abdomen, no matter your type. In addition to triggering abdominal fat gain, smoking causes a host of other ill effects—raising your risk of cancer, heart disease, and other health problems. For these reasons, I recommend that all types refrain from smoking.

Keep control of alcohol. The research is clear: Too much alcohol does indeed lead to a beer belly! I recommend that all types hold their alcohol consumption to one drink or fewer a day. While on phases 1 and 2 of the eating plan, I recommend you drink no alcohol, as it may unravel your resolve to stick to the meal plan.

If you are a sedentary person who routinely skimps on sleep, eats an unhealthy diet, and is exposed to a lot of stress, it may seem like a lot to change at once. The good news is you don't have to do everything at once! Although in the ideal world you would do everything right—sleeping well, eating well, relaxing, exercising, the works—I know you have a real life with real commitments. That's why I developed this plan. It will show you what's most important for you to tackle first, in the real world, based on your tummy type, to get the results you deserve—and quickly.

Now let's turn to Chapter 3 to discover your tummy type!

PART TWO

WHAT'S YOUR TUMMY TYPE?

3 YOUR TUMMY TYPE

Take This Simple Quiz and Then Turn to the Corresponding Chapter to Discover Your Unique Solution to Slimming Down

I don't know about you, but I love taking simple quizzes. I see them as a fun opportunity to learn more about myself. The quiz outlined in the following pages is no different; it will ask you a specific set of questions that will help you to determine your personal tummy type. Once you know your type, you can turn to the chapter that features your own tummy type (Chapters 4 through 9) to discover the solution that will work most effectively for you.

In the following quiz, you will be asked some questions that may require you to seek guidance from your family doctor. To accurately determine your tummy type, you will need to know your waist measurement, hip measurement, height, weight, blood pressure, cholesterol profile, and blood sugar level. Your doctor can do a simple blood test to help you determine some of that information. I always recommend that people who are about to start an exercise program first check with their doctors; consider this a bit of extra incentive! Plus, I'm a big believer in an annual checkup. I do a full physical with an internist every year. And, of course, if you're eager to start and you have this data from a recent visit, you can certainly use it to determine your tummy type, as most people's type tends to remain the same—until they find a solution to change it!

As you complete the self-assessment, check the corresponding box in the chart (on page 34) under the letter that best describes your answer. If you are a man, assessing your type is easy. You can simply turn to Chapter 9 to find out everything you need to know about your type.

1. **What is your body mass index?**

   Your body mass index (BMI) is a number derived from your weight and height. To determine your BMI, divide your weight in pounds by your height in inches squared, then multiply the resulting number by 703. For example, if you weigh 150 pounds and stand 5 feet 5 inches tall, you would calculate your BMI as follows:

   $$[150 \div (65 \times 65)] \times 703 = 24.96$$

   If you're simply not a math person and the formula above makes your head ache, the following government-run trustworthy Web sites will calculate your BMI for you.

   www.cdc.gov/nccdphp/dnpa/bmi/index.htm

   http://nhlbisupport.com/bmi/

   A body mass index below 18.5 is considered underweight; between 18.5 and 24.9, normal weight; and 25 or above, overweight or obese. If your BMI is 24.9 or less, check off "D" in the box that corresponds to question #1. If it is 25 or above, leave this box blank.

2. **What is the circumference of your waist in inches?**

   Measure the smallest part of your waist without sucking in your tummy. A waist measurement above 35 inches could qualify you as any of the tummy types. So place a check mark in the chart for all of the lettered boxes if your waist measures 35 inches or more. Check no boxes if it measures less than 35 inches. I included this question because a waist measurement of 35 inches or more for women (and 40 for men) is strongly associated with an increased risk of heart disease and poor health. So your answer to this question should give you even more incentive to stick with this program!

3. **What is your waist-to-hip ratio?**

   Your waist-to-hip ratio (WHR) helps to pinpoint how you store your excess weight: all over your body, mostly in the hips, or mostly in the tummy. In practical terms, a woman with equal waist and hip measurements of 34 inches would have a 1:1 ratio, signifying a high waist-to-hip ratio. Women with high waist-to-hip ratios are often referred to as apple shaped, as opposed to women with low WHRs, who are referred to as pear shaped.

To determine your waist-to-hip ratio, measure around the smallest part of your waistline. Then measure your hips at the widest point. Divide your waist measurement by your hip measurement. Prevention.com has an online calculator that will do this math for you: www.prevention.com/bmicalculator.

If your waist-to-hip ratio is 0.8 or above, check off A, B, and D in the chart. If it is below 0.8, leave the boxes for this question blank.

4. **What is your HDL cholesterol level?**

   If your HDL cholesterol reading is less than 50 milligrams per deciliter (mg/dl), place a check mark under B in the box that corresponds to this question. If it is 50 mg/dl or more, leave the boxes that correspond to this question blank.

5. **What is your triglyceride level?**

   If your fasting plasma triglyceride level is 150 mg/dl or greater, check off B for this question. If it is less than 150 mg/dl, leave the boxes that correspond to this question blank.

6. **What is your fasting blood glucose level?**

   If it is 110 mg/dl or more, check off B for this question. If it is less than 110 mg/dl, leave the boxes that correspond to this question blank.

7. **What is your blood pressure?**

   If your usual blood pressure reading is 130/85 millimeters of mercury (mm Hg) or higher, check off B for this question. If it is less than 130/85 mm Hg, leave the boxes that correspond to this question blank.

8. **Have you stopped menstruating due to menopause?**

   If you answered yes, check off C for this question. If you answered no, check no boxes.

9. **Have you gained weight in your tummy your entire life—even as far back as high school?**

   If you answered yes, check off A for this question. If you answered no, check no boxes.

10. **Are you older than age 40 and noticed that your body shape is starting to change, causing you to gain fat in your tummy—a place you never before gained it?**

    If you answered yes, check C for this question. Otherwise, check no boxes.

11. **If you are postmenopausal, have you gained 5 or more pounds—mostly in your tummy—during "the change"?**

    If you answered yes, check C for this question. Otherwise, check no boxes.

12. **Do you feel that there is too much stress in your life?**

    If you answered yes, check D in the box that corresponds to this question. If you answered no, check no boxes.

13. **Have you been fairly slender most of your life but noticed your tummy starting to get poochy when you changed jobs, bought a new home, started planning a wedding, or experienced some other stressful life event?**

    If you answered yes, check D for this question. If you answered no, leave this question blank.

14. **Did you feel confident about your tummy until you had a baby?**

    If you answered yes, check E for this question. If you answered no, check no boxes.

15. **Have you given birth to a baby within the past 2 years?**

    If you answered yes, check E for this question. If you answered no, check no boxes.

Type Chart

Check off the box under each letter that corresponds to your answers to each quiz question and then add up your answers in each column.

	A	B	C	D	E
1					
2					
3					
4					
5					
6					

	A	**B**	**C**	**D**	**E**
7					
8					
9					
10					
11					
12					
13					
14					
15					
Totals					

Answer Key

The most check marks for any one letter will determine your tummy type. If you have the same or nearly the same amount of check marks for two or more letters, this simply means that you may be a borderline type. For example, you may be a genetic apple who recently had a baby. In this case, read the chapters for both types and determine, based on what you learn, which type most specifically describes your situation today.

Below you will find your tummy type according to the letter you most checked in the quiz, along with the corresponding chapter to turn to for more information.

A. Apple Type, Chapter 4

B. Metabolically Challenged Type, Chapter 5

C. Peri/Postmenopause Type, Chapter 6

D. Stressed Slender Type, Chapter 7

E. After Baby Type, Chapter 8

While many of you will find it impossible to resist looking at *your* chapter first—and really, why fight it?—I encourage you to read the other tummy types' chapters as well. You may gain information that will help you at a different stage in your life, or perhaps you'll pick up some tidbit of helpful information for a girlfriend, your mom, or someone else you love. Knowledge is powerful—just like a strong and firm tummy!

4 THE APPLE TYPE

Genetics Has Caused You to Store Excess Fat in Your Tummy Most of Your Adult Life

For many years scientists have split women into two categories: apples and pears. The pears tend to gain weight in their hips and thighs, whereas the apples tend to gain weight in their breasts, arms, and tummies. Apples have slender legs and small rear ends but tend to have large breasts and round tummies. Although some pears turn into apples after menopause, you're only a true apple if you've gained weight in your tummy—and not in your hips or thighs—as far back as you can remember.

You can blame 30 to 60 percent of your body shape on your genetics. Unfortunately, the excess fat you store in your tummy raises your risk for developing heart disease, type 2 diabetes, and breast and uterine cancers. The good news, however, is that your specific body type may allow you to lose this fat more easily than other types can. And losing just 2 inches around your waist can lower your risk for these diseases by 50 to 60 percent!

To trim your midsection, you will focus on lifestyle changes that reduce levels of the hormone testosterone. Although we tend to think of testosterone as a male hormone and progesterone and estrogen as female hormones, both sexes produce these hormones in differing amounts. Most women produce some testosterone in small amounts, but one of the main reasons you tend to gain weight in your tummy is that you produce higher-than-usual levels of this typically male hormone. Your body may also produce lower-than-normal levels of the female hormones estrogen and progesterone, making menstruation somewhat erratic and possibly even hindering your fertility.

TONE YOUR APPLE TUMMY

While everyone will get great results using the Core Diet and Core Moves (which start on page 83 and page 95, respectively), an Apple Tummy Type can get even more impressive results by focusing on these key strategies, developed to tap into and make the most of her particular biochemistry.

TOP TUMMY TACTIC **1. Hit the streets.** The most immediate, effective thing you can do to trim your tummy is to get a bit more cardio exercise than is recommended in the Core Moves plan. Endurance exercise helps to reduce testosterone levels, so adding some extra can have a big impact on your silhouette almost immediately. In addition to the routines recommended in the fitness plan, add a daily power walk (or run) of 20 minutes or longer. Also, when you do your exercise routines, use lighter weights and perform more than the suggested number of repetitions at a fast cadence. This will help to boost your heart rate during these routines to drive down testosterone even more.

2. Take a daily time-out. High levels of stress tax your adrenal glands, which respond by raising testosterone levels. If you're one of those on-the-go types who never takes time to smell the roses, incorporate a time-out into your day. You can do anything during this 5- to 10-minute break as long as you don't find it stressful. Listen to soft music, sit quietly as you breathe deeply, do a few yoga moves, or go for a short walk. Do what works for you to calm down and refocus.

3. Get a checkup. Apple types have a higher risk of developing a condition called polycystic ovarian syndrome, which is characterized by high testosterone levels and insulin resistance (which means that your cells do not respond normally to this hormone). In addition to hindering your fertility, this health condition can trigger the growth of excess body hair. Successful treatment will improve these symptoms as well as help you lose that tummy fat.

4. Always eat some protein with meals and snacks. In addition to higher-than-usual levels of the hormone testosterone, apple types tend to have elevated levels of the hormone insulin. These levels will come down somewhat as you get in shape and lose weight. In the meantime, you can balance insulin levels by avoiding any meal or snack composed of pure carbohydrate. For example, never have toast with jam. A better snack for you is toast with peanut butter. Similarly, rather than pasta with tomato sauce only, you'll want to include some lean turkey meatballs.

The Apple's Top Tummy-Slimming Snack

Emerging research shows that the mineral calcium—particularly when consumed from dairy products—can help burn tummy fat. As a genetic apple, you're fighting one of the toughest battles against tummy fat and need to use every tummy-slimming strategy available. That's why I made sure that your tummy-slimming snack contains plenty of this important tummy-slimming mineral. The following Maple Ricotta Spread snack recipe includes plenty of this bone-building and fat-burning mineral. To make it, mix ⅓ cup fat-free ricotta cheese with 1 tablespoon maple syrup and 1 teaspoon brown sugar. Spread it over a slice of whole grain toast or a whole grain waffle, or use it as a dip for 4 graham cracker squares. Feel free to substitute this snack for other snacks called for on the Core Diet plan.

The Apple's Top Three Moves

In addition to your routines described in Chapter 11, do the following three moves every day to boost your heart rate. I suggest you do them in the morning to get your heart rate up right away. It only takes a few minutes to complete, but your metabolism will remain elevated for some time afterward. For extra credit, do the routine a few additional times during the day when you want to rev up your energy. Take a break midmorning or mid-afternoon for a set. Or, to blast away the stress of the day, try it right after work. You can do the routine either barefoot (if you're doing it on a carpeted surface) or with shoes. This extra cardio will help to drive down testosterone levels.

I TONED MY TUMMY!

MEGAN MCGINNIS
TUMMY TYPE: **Apple**
AGE: **22**
HOMETOWN: **New York, New York**
RESULTS: **Lost 6 pounds and 2 inches from her tummy area in 4 weeks**
LIFE-CHANGING EXPERIENCE: **Became happier and healthier**

When my mom found out she had diabetes, it was a major wake-up call. I realized that my weight is about much more than my appearance and that if I didn't start eating right and exercising consistently, there would be serious consequences for me in the future.

Over the years, I gained weight for a combination of reasons. I grew up with unhealthy eating habits. My parents went out to eat constantly, so I continued to do the same through college and after I graduated. When I ate out, not only did I make bad choices, the portions were huge! I was also not good at sticking to a set exercise routine. I would go to the gym regularly for a few months, and then school or work would become stressful and get in the way. When I stopped exercising, my eating habits would also worsen.

Two years ago, I lost 20 pounds, and my stomach became flat. I felt great! Then I gained it all back, which tarnished my self-esteem. I felt terrible about myself and stopped caring about how I looked.

I decided to start Denise Austin's Tone Your Tummy Type program in an effort to boost my self-esteem, improve my appearance, and, most important, become healthier. Four weeks into the program, I am so happy I decided to participate. I love the eating plan—the food is both delicious and easy to prepare. I don't have a lot of spare time or cooking skills, but I am still able to make the recipes with ease. My boyfriend has also tried some of the foods and likes them as well.

The cardio routine in the program is fun to do and requires minimal equipment, which is nice. I turn on the radio and do the exercises to music.

Overall, after adopting the healthier eating and exercise habits on Denise's Tone Your Tummy Type program, I feel wonderful—so much better! I can see the difference in my body, and so can my boyfriend—he says my stomach looks more toned. As I see the pounds coming off, I am more and more motivated to lose additional inches and pounds. Thanks, Denise!

KNEE BEND WITH OVERHEAD REACH

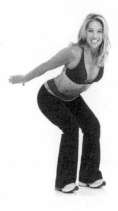

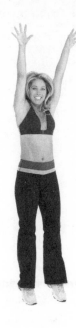

A

B

Stand with your feet under your hips. All in one motion, bend your knees and sit back into a squat as you lower your arms.

Then straighten your legs as you raise your arms overhead. If you're up to it first thing in the morning, throw in a jump, as shown, into the air before landing and completing another squat. Repeat for a total of 10 to 15 times. Do this movement quickly. Your goal is to boost metabolism.

JUMPING JACKS

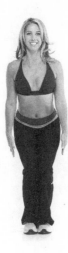

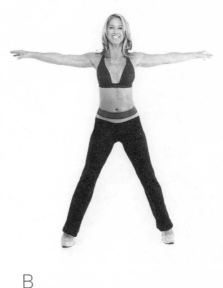

A

Start with your feet under your hips and arms at your sides.

B

Jump your feet out to the sides into a wide angle as you simultaneously lift your arms laterally out to the sides. Jump back in as you lower your arms. Repeat for 1 minute.

ELBOW STRIKE AND JAB

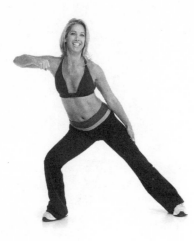

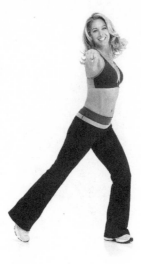

A

Stand with your feet under your hips. Step to the side with your right leg, bending your right knee and sitting back into your right buttocks as you simultaneously swing your right elbow back behind, as if you were trying to strike someone behind you with your elbow.

B

Then shift your body weight onto your left leg, bending your left knee as you straighten your right leg and rise onto the ball of your right foot. Throw a punch with your right arm, as if you were trying to hit someone standing directly in front of you, as shown. Continue to alternate elbow strikes and jabs with your right arm for 30 seconds. Then switch to your left side.

5 THE METABOLICALLY CHALLENGED TYPE

A Precursor to Diabetes, Your Insulin-Resistant
State Can Be Reversed with Diet and Exercise

If your quiz results place you in this tummy type, you either have or are developing a condition called metabolic syndrome. Your muscle cells don't respond normally to the hormone insulin, requiring your pancreas to secrete unusually high amounts of it to shuttle sugar out of your blood and into cells that can burn it for energy. Characterized by high blood cholesterol, high blood pressure, increased levels of fasting blood sugar, and, of course, tummy fat, this health condition raises your risk for a number of diseases.

You probably have not been metabolically challenged your entire life. When you were younger, your metabolism may have functioned normally. With age, however, the hormone insulin tends to lose its effectiveness. Both age and hormonal changes at menopause increase your risk of metabolic syndrome. Indeed, 47 percent of postmenopausal women have this condition.

The Tone Your Tummy Type Core Diet and Core Moves plans are

especially well suited for your tummy type. The inflammation-lowering diet, for example, is low in saturated fat and added sugars, both of which will help you to reduce your risk of heart disease and improve your insulin sensitivity (so cells take up sugar more readily). Some experts believe that eating too much of the wrong types of fat causes *90 percent* of type 2 diabetes cases (and metabolic syndrome often leads to diabetes). Saturated fat is associated with tummy fat, especially the dangerous, deep visceral type. The Tone Your Tummy Type Core Diet will help you to decrease the bad fats and boost levels of good fats to calm metabolic syndrome.

Think about it this way: The metabolic syndrome is your early-warning system. I always say that if you're diagnosed with metabolic syndrome, you should consider it a blessing—you still have a chance to make changes that can have a great impact on your long-term health and your life span. Please take this condition very seriously; without your efforts to lose weight and get fit, these conditions tend to reinforce each other, and you might find yourself in a tricky downward spiral, healthwise. And I care about you too much to see that happen!

The most exciting line of research for your tummy type shows that proper diet and enough exercise may be the only changes you need to make to reverse this condition, helping you to shrink your tummy and reduce your blood pressure, blood cholesterol, and blood sugar and insulin levels. In fact, one study determined that these lifestyle changes may work as effectively as the diabetes drug metformin at reversing metabolic syndrome. Follow your tummy type program, and you'll start walking far away from this sneaky syndrome.

TONE YOUR METABOLICALLY CHALLENGED TUMMY

While everyone will get great results using the Core Diet and Core Moves (which start on page 83 and page 95, respectively), a Metabolically Challenged Tummy Type can get even more impressive results by focusing on these key strategies, developed to tap into and make the most of her particular biochemistry.

TOP TUMMY TACTIC | **1. Pick up the intensity during your workouts.** According to a study of 6,000 women that spanned 9 years at Northwestern Memorial Hospital in Chicago, women who were diagnosed with metabolic syndrome were 57 percent more likely to die within that period than women who did not have this syndrome. Before you let that statistic scare you, however, listen to this piece of good news: Women with metabolic syndrome who were aerobically fit had the same risk of death as women who did not have the condition. What is a high level of aerobic fitness? The Northwestern Memorial Hospital researchers defined it as being able to run a mile in 12 minutes or faster. So if you currently walk for fitness, pick up the pace, doing bursts of faster walking or running during your normal session. For example, for every 3 minutes of walking, add a minute of faster walking or jogging. If you can't or don't like to run, do the same interval workout during any activity. Try it while swimming, cycling, or doing any other non-weight-bearing activity. Push yourself! You can do it.

2. Reduce processed and sugary carbs. The Tone Your Tummy Type Core Diet plan includes very few processed and sugary carbohydrates. Follow the meal plan closely in this regard, as high amounts of added sugars or processed carbs (white bread, snack crackers, and any food made from white flour) tend to raise blood sugar levels, which in turn raise insulin levels and trigger insulin resistance.

3. Rein in sodium. People with metabolic syndrome tend to absorb more sodium from their food than people who do not have this syndrome. Not only can this bloat your tummy, the high sodium levels also raise blood pressure. Do not salt your food, and please try to wean yourself off high-sodium foods such as processed foods, fast food (see strategy #4), and canned soup.

4. Adopt a slow-food lifestyle. Research completed by many institutions and funded by the National Heart, Lung, and Blood Institute has found that people who eat fast food more than twice a week gained an extra 10 pounds and were two times as likely to develop insulin resistance (which leads to metabolic syndrome) over 15 years than people who ate fast food less than once a week.

The Metabolically Challenged's Top Tummy-Slimming Snack

The following snack is loaded with health-promoting monounsaturated fats, which will help protect your heart and extend your life—both important goals when you have metabolic syndrome. It also contains a moderate amount of protein to stabilize blood sugar levels. Feel free to substitute this snack for any snack listed on your meal plan. To make the Crunchy Cottage Cheese Bowl, top ¾ cup 1% fat or fat-free cottage cheese with 2 tablespoons low-fat granola cereal and 1 tablespoon sunflower seeds.

I TONED MY TUMMY!

RAMONA RAE

TUMMY TYPE: **Metabolically Challenged**

AGE: **48**

HOMETOWN: **St. George, Utah**

RESULTS: **Lost 7 pounds and 2 inches from her waist in 4 weeks**

LIFE-CHANGING EXPERIENCE: **Reduced her daily insulin intake**

For my 45th birthday, I got a very unwanted gift—20 pounds. Without changing anything in my diet or activity level, I gained 5 pounds each month in the 4 months following my birthday.

I suspect some of the "birthday 20" was the result of my having diabetes. I've never had a flat tummy, but my stomach really grew when I started to take insulin. Before Denise Austin's Tone Your Tummy Type program, I hadn't been able to get rid of my tummy. It was really frustrating—I felt totally helpless!

When the opportunity arose to try Denise's program, I decided to go for it for a few different reasons. For one, I was unhappy with my appearance. I hated looking in the mirror, buying clothes, or even getting dressed in the morning because I didn't think I looked good. The second and more important reason was my health. In addition to the diabetes, I struggle with high cholesterol and high blood pressure, and I wanted to do something to improve those numbers. It was the perfect time for me to change my diet, my exercise habits, and the overall shape of my body.

Four weeks into the program, I can feel that my stomach muscles are stronger. I now know that cardiovascular exercise and a lower-fat diet really do lead to weight loss, particularly in the tummy region.

Best of all, I've been able to reduce my daily insulin amount and have my blood sugar levels under better control. I attribute this to the healthful, high-fiber foods in Denise's plan.

Overall, I feel much better about myself and more confident in my appearance. I no longer dread getting dressed in the morning; in fact, I look forward to it! I am truly grateful for the Tone Your Tummy Type program, and I can't wait to see even more results as I continue the program in the future.

The Metabolically Challenged's Top Three Moves

The higher your level of fitness, the more efficiently your muscles will burn sugar for energy, which will help keep insulin levels low. Your exercise routines will help you to improve your fitness. To speed up your results, do the following three moves every day for only a few minutes. Think of them as extra credit. They will help you challenge your muscles just that much more in only a few extra minutes. The following traditional movements will strengthen the muscles in your chest, arms, abs, shoulders, and legs. That's quite effective for just three movements! You can do them barefoot or with shoes. I suggest you do them first thing in the morning so that you're sure to fit them in, ensuring that you get that extra exercise boost. They will help you to build the muscle needed to keep insulin levels in check all day long.

PUSHUP

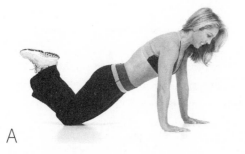

A

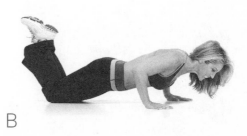

B

This is a great strength-building move for your upper body. Kneel and place your palms on the floor so that your body forms a straight line from your knees to your head.

Bend your elbows out to the sides as you lower your chest to the floor, keeping your abdomen firm and your back flat. Lift to the starting position and repeat for a total of 8 to 12 times. *Note:* You can do this exercise with your legs extended to increase the challenge.

HIP CIRCLES AND WAIST TRIMMERS

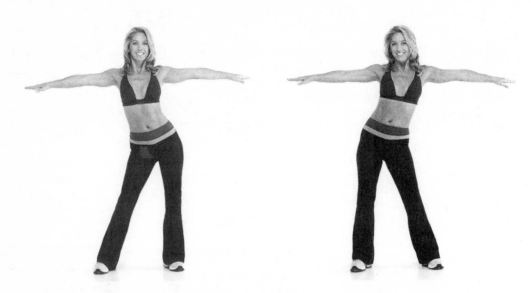

A

Stand with your feel slightly wider than your hips. Soften your knees, allowing a very slight bend. Extend your arms at shoulder height from your sides. Firm your tummy and circle your hips, starting by sticking your left hip out to the left as far as you can.

B

Try to use only your tummy muscles to bring your hips in a circle, pressing your buttocks back and then your hips to the right, as shown, and then front. Circle for 30 seconds in this counterclockwise direction. Then switch direction and circle for another 30 seconds.

WARRIOR II

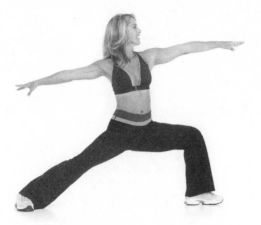

This is great for your hips, thighs, and buttocks. Stand with your legs in a wide angle.
Turn your left foot out 90 degrees and slide
your right heel out slightly. Lift your arms
out to the sides to shoulder level. Lift up
through your abdominals, tuck your tailbone
slightly, and bend your left knee up to 90
degrees. Hold for 30 seconds. Rise and
repeat on the other side.

6 THE PERI/POST-MENOPAUSE TYPE

Falling Hormone Levels Signal Tummy Fat Cells to Fill Up

About two-thirds of women gain weight as they approach menopause or just after menopause—usually in their tummies. Even friends of mine who had naturally flat tummies in their youth now tell me that their tummies are no longer their best feature. Indeed, it's during perimenopause (the time leading up to the cessation of your cycle) that many women tell me their tried-and-true exercise-and-diet plan just no longer works.

Before I explain how to turn things around, I first want you to understand what is going on inside your body. As your menstrual cycles come to a halt, your levels of the female sex hormone estrogen start to fall. Levels of the male hormone testosterone may fall as well, but not as dramatically as estrogen, causing you to exhibit a more male-pattern body type with a big middle but relatively slender thighs and hips. At the same time, levels of the stress hormone cortisol rise after menopause, which also contributes to fat gain in the abdomen. Your metabolic rate also slows down, causing you to gain weight, even though you are not overeating or underexercising.

Many women, like myself, notice a change in their tummy type before any other menopausal symptom. I still menstruate regularly and have no hot flashes or other hallmarks of menopause. Yet, I know my hormonal levels are switching because I more easily gain weight in my tummy.

In years past many physicians considered synthetic estrogen and progesterone a fountain of youth for women during perimenopause and after menopause. Subsequent research, however, has linked hormone therapy (HT) with an increased risk of heart disease and breast cancer. Also, other research shows that taking these drugs may not as effectively reduce abdominal fat gain as once thought. For these reasons, I suggest you carefully weigh the pros and cons of HT, getting plenty of input from your family physician and gynecologist before making a decision.

If you decide to forgo HT (or even if you decide to take HT), there are plenty of natural ways to shrink belly fat. Don't despair! You do not have to accept a few extra pounds around the middle as a rite of passage.

TONE YOUR PERI/POSTMENOPAUSE TUMMY

While everyone will get great results using the Core Diet and Core Moves (which start on page 83 and page 95, respectively), a Peri/Postmenopause Tummy Type can get even more impressive results by focusing on these key strategies, developed to tap into and make the most of her particular biochemistry.

TOP TUMMY TACTIC **1. Aim for 45.** Forty-five minutes of exercise, that is, 5 days a week. In addition to reducing your risk of cancer and heart disease (which rise after menopause), studies done at the Fred Hutchinson Cancer Research Center in Seattle show that moderate exercise (especially if you've been sedentary) effectively reduces abdominal fat after menopause. This yearlong study of 170 sedentary, postmenopausal women showed that moderate-intensity exercise shrunk their abdominal fat by between 3.4 percent and 6.9 percent, even though they had continued to eat the same amount of daily calories. Women who stretched but did not exercise gained abdominal fat.

Your exercise routines in Chapter 11 will only satisfy about half of your daily exercise goal. In addition to those routines, add 20 to 25 minutes of power walking (or another

I TONED MY TUMMY!

SUE KEILITZ

TUMMY TYPE: **Peri/Postmenopause**

AGE: **63**

HOMETOWN: **Mount Pleasant, Michigan**

RESULTS: **Lost 8½ pounds and 4 inches from her waist (15 inches total off her body!) in 4 weeks**

LIFE-CHANGING EXPERIENCE: **Decided to start living life to the fullest**

When my mother passed away last December, I was devastated. She was my best friend. After her death, I decided to become the best person I could. I wanted to live my life as she had lived hers. I learned to play the piano (Mom was self-taught), and I vowed to lose weight and become stronger with exercise.

Tone Your Tummy Type was the perfect program to help me lose weight because tummy fat has been a part of my life for as long as I can remember. Even when I was a teenager, I carried around a spare tire either above or below my waist (usually both places). My mother and sister had the exact same tummy, so I guess it is partially hereditary.

I attribute my tummy fat to a few things. For one, although I've used Denise Austin's exercise videos for a while, I wasn't using them nearly often enough, and I lived an otherwise sedentary lifestyle.

Second, I love sweets and (used to!) eat a lot of them. When I read Denise's paragraph stating that sugar is the worst thing for tummy fat, I had mixed emotions. I was surprised, but at the same time, I was pleased to know that I could do something about my tummy—my genes didn't completely dictate how my tummy looked!

Tone Your Tummy Type is an amazing program. After only 1 week, I had lost 4½ pounds, 1½ inches off my waist, 2 inches off my hips, 1½ inches off my thighs, 1½ inches off my bust, and ½ inch off my upper arms. I couldn't believe it!

I did not feel like I had to sacrifice for these instant results. I am never hungry on the program, and it is such a joy to prepare the recipes. I have tried so many different foods I'd never eaten before. The herbs and spices add so much flavor to the recipes that I never miss the added salt or sugar.

Since I started Denise's program, my energy level has been amazing! I can go all day—ride my bike and play with my four granddaughters. I am thankful for the opportunity to participate in the Tone Your Tummy Type trial program. I am thrilled with my results, and I know my mom would be very proud.

type of cardiovascular exercise) to your day. If you would rather get all of your cardio out of the way at once, lengthen the cardio segments of the Core Cardio Blast routine described in Chapter 11, making each cardio segment last for 7 minutes.

2. Consider taking a meditation class. Meditation has been shown to increase levels of dehydroepiandrosterone (DHEA), a hormone produced in the adrenal glands that—in optimal levels—improves insulin sensitivity *and* reduces abdominal fat. Your adrenal glands produce less DHEA as you age. The exercise you will complete on the Tone Your Tummy Type plan will also help bolster levels of this natural hormone.

3. Eat 7 to 10 servings of vegetables and fruits day. High intakes of vegetables and fruits protect your bone and heart health after menopause. In terms of shrinking tummy fat, I like to champion vegetables in particular. They are high in fiber and water—which helps fill you up—but very low in calories. After menopause, as your metabolism slows, you'll need to eat fewer calories. Adding more vegetables helps you to eat fewer calories without resorting to eating a smaller volume of food. To achieve this ideal level, eat two produce servings with each of your three main meals and add in a couple as snacks between meals. The Tone Your Tummy Type Core Diet menus include—on average—six servings of fruits and vegetables a day. So, you need only add one additional serving of vegetables to meet this quota. ("More food?" you're thinking. "Okay!")

4. Relax—daily. Stress interferes with the functioning of your adrenal glands. You need these glands to function effectively after menopause, as they assist in the production of estrogen by your fat cells. Whenever you begin to feel anxious, jittery, or tense, stop what you are doing. Close your eyes (if possible) and focus on your breathing. Try to take deep breaths from your tummy, in and out slowly through your nose. If you still can't relax, try tensing and then—on the exhale—releasing the muscles in your body. Start with your feet and move up to your heart. Then, try to tense your entire body at once and release as you sigh. You'll feel relaxed and clearheaded.

5. Take a fiber supplement. Your metabolism slows at menopause, meaning you'll need to eat about 200 fewer calories to prevent weight gain. A fiber supplement such as Benefiber will help reduce hunger, allowing you to eat less without feeling hungry.

The Peri/Postmenopause's Top Tummy-Slimming Snack

My Berry Flax Smoothie contains a wealth of omega-3 fats (important for fighting inflammation) and antioxidants that will help you to prevent heart disease, cancer, and other diseases that tend to become common after menopause. It also tastes sweet, allowing you to indulge in a sweet, refreshing, and healthful treat without derailing your weight-loss goals. In a blender, combine 2 cups fresh or unsweetened, frozen raspberries; 4 tablespoons calcium-fortified orange juice; 6 ounces fat-free French Vanilla Stonyfield Farm yogurt; 1 tablespoon flax meal or flaxseeds; and 1 tablespoon wheat germ. Blend until smooth.

The Peri/Postmenopause's Top Three Moves

To help you meet your daily 45 minutes of cardiovascular exercise, try the following fun dance routine first thing each morning to ensure you fit it in. It's a great way to greet the day with a smile! You can do it with shoes or barefoot. If you enjoy the moves, also consider doing it a few additional times a day to add up those cardio minutes. Try it as a morning or afternoon break. Or do it right after work to help transition your mind to home life. Put on some music and dance. It's a great way to get moving in a healthy way!

CHASSÉ INTO ROCK STEPS

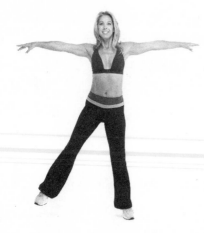 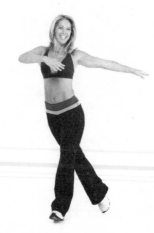

A

Starting with your feet under your hips, take a shuffle step laterally to the left, using your right foot to chase your left out of position.

B

Then plant your left foot and take a step back and to the left with your right foot. Step your feet back into the same plane and then shuffle to the right, this time stepping back with the left foot. Continue shuffling back and forth for 1 minute.

What's Your Tummy Type?

STEP TOUCHES

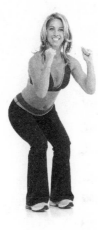

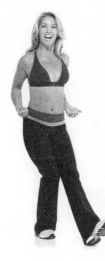

A

B

Stand with your feet under your hips. Bend your elbows and lift your hands to shoulder level. Bend your knees and squat down slightly.

Step forward with your right leg, tapping the floor with your heel. As you step out, pull your elbows behind you. Step your feet back together and then step forward with your left leg, as shown. Continue alternating legs for 1 minute.

CHA-CHA

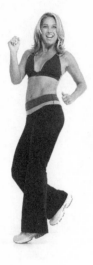

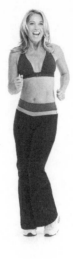

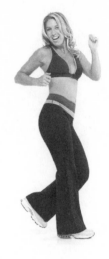

A

Start with your feet under your hips. Step forward and slightly to the right with your left foot, swiveling your hips as you do so, as shown.

B

Step your feet back under your hips, swiveling them again to a "cha cha cha" cadence.

C

Then step forward and slightly to the left. Do the cha-cha for 1 minute.

7 THE STRESSED SLENDER TYPE

High Cortisol Levels Shuttle Fat into That Small Potbelly

When you complain about your tummy, your friends probably tease you, saying that they wish their tummies looked like yours. Indeed, if you're a true stressed slender type, you don't wage a global battle with body fat. You like your arms, legs, and tush. Your tummy is just rounder and flabbier than you'd prefer, despite your stellar exercise and eating habits.

Why is your tummy so round when the rest of you is so slender? In a word: stress. Stress activates the fight-or-flight response, the body's answer to a threatening situation. This response makes your heart pound and your breath shorten. During the fight-or-flight response, the body releases the stress hormone cortisol, which, among other things, bolsters your appetite for sweets and simple carbohydrate foods. Researchers have long known that people with diseases that cause extreme exposure to the stress hormone cortisol (such as Cushing's syndrome) tend to have high amounts of abdominal fat. When cortisol is high, abdominal fat cells increase in size.

Research completed at Yale University shows that lean women may be more vulnerable to the effects of stress than heavier women are. In other words, when you're a thin woman caught in traffic or under a deadline at work, you secrete more cortisol than another woman with a few more pounds who might be caught in the same stressful situation. You also may have difficulty adapting to stress. Whereas some people feel anxious the first time they face a difficult situation—but then develop coping skills to adapt—you may feel off center every single time you face a given situation.

As a result, you are more likely than other women to see the effects of stress in your tummy. The Tone Your Tummy Type Core Diet—which is low in added sugars and processed carbohydrates—will help to calm your nervous system. The Core Moves plan will help to bolster levels of calming, feel-good chemicals, called endorphins, in your brain. Other research completed at Yale shows that just 10 minutes of vigorous exercise is all you need to trigger this calming endorphin response.

TONE YOUR STRESSED SLENDER TUMMY

While everyone will get great results using the Core Diet and Core Moves (which start on page 83 and page 95 respectively), a Stressed Slender Tummy Type can get even more impressive results by focusing on these key strategies, developed to tap into and make the most of her particular biochemistry.

TOP TUMMY TACTIC | **1. Carve out "me" time.** One or two times a day (two is ideal), designate 15 to 20 minutes to relax. Turn off the phone, pager, cell phone, e-mail, and other distractions. Lie in a comfortable position on the floor or sit in a comfortable chair. Close your eyes and take 3 deep breaths, imagining yourself exhaling all of your tension. Then, breathing normally, systematically relax your muscles, starting at your feet and working up to your head. First, tense each muscle area as you inhale, and then release that tension as you exhale. Tense and release your feet, legs, buttocks, abdomen and back, arms, shoulders, neck, and face. Then rest comfortably for a few moments, noticing how relaxation feels. Over time and with enough practice, you'll be able to cultivate this sense of relaxation within seconds whenever you start to feel stressed.

2. Eat frequent meals. Hunger is a stressor on the body that can trigger the release of cortisol. The Tone Your Tummy Type Core Diet plan calls for a daily snack, which will

I TONED MY TUMMY!

ROBIN RYE

TUMMY TYPE: **Stressed Slender**

AGE: **45**

HOMETOWN: **Galt, California**

RESULTS: **Lost 4 pounds and 1½ inches from her tummy area in 4 weeks**

LIFE-CHANGING EXPERIENCE: **Got rid of her heartburn and looks forward to exercise**

I never had to worry about my weight—in fact, I was underweight until I hit 30. Life eventually started to catch up with me, however, and the pounds did start to pile on in my tummy for a number of reasons.

One, I never really lost all the weight from my two pregnancies. Then, during the last few years, my son became ill with a series of bone infections, my mother died from Alzheimer's disease, and my cousin died after a 2-year battle with cancer. On top of all that, my father has recently developed health problems that require a great deal of my help and support. All the stress in my life left me with a spare tire that I couldn't get rid of, that is, until I started Denise Austin's Tone Your Tummy Type program.

I decided to participate in the Tone Your Tummy Type trial because my weight was taking a real toll on my self-esteem and health. I avoided swimming because I didn't want to be seen in a bathing suit, and I developed high blood pressure and heartburn. I was down, mentally and physically, and I decided it was time to turn things around.

So far, Denise's program has worked quite well for me and helped me to lose 4 pounds and 1½ inches around my waist.

The recipes are delicious, and they give me the peace of mind of knowing I'm always getting the right balance of carbohydrates and protein. Because I'm eating well, I feel more energetic and I *want* to do the exercises.

The movements in the program have taught me to properly work my abs for maximum results, and I genuinely look forward to doing them.

Best of all, I feel wonderful physically. As I approach menopause, I feel more prepared than before to ward off health problems I may face at this stage of my life. I have more energy to go on bike rides with my boys and to play ball at the park. My heartburn has gone away since I started the program. The Tone Your Tummy Type program has been great for my husband and kids as well. My husband has been eating some of the recipes, and his blood sugar levels are under better control. It has been a wonderful transformation for us all. Thanks so much!

help. Consider splitting this daily snack in two, eating part of it in the morning and part in the midafternoon to quell hunger.

3. Do the right amount of exercise for your fitness level. Too much exercise will further stress your system, raising cortisol levels. So start slowly, listening to how you feel. If the exercise routines feel too hard, ease up. You might, for example, stick with the phase 1 routines longer than 2 weeks before ramping up to phase 2.

4. Go to bed and wake up at the same time every day. Chronic sleep deprivation can raise cortisol levels. When you go to bed and awaken at the same time each day, you give your body the cues it needs to fall asleep quickly, stay asleep, and wake feeling refreshed. When you follow a haphazard sleep schedule, you'll find that you toss and turn more often. I recommend you hit the sack and wake up at the same time even on weekends as you do during the week.

5. Watch funny movies on a regular basis. Now, this is a tactic anyone can stick with! In a study conducted at the Loma Linda University Center for Neuroimmunology in California, participants who watched a humorous video had 30 percent less cortisol in their blood during and after watching the tape than other participants who did not watch the video.

The Stressed Slender's Top Tummy-Slimming Snack

Crunchy foods help dissipate stress, which is probably why so many people turn to potato chips and pretzels when they feel stressed. The following Vegetable and Onion Dip includes lots of crunchy vegetables—a whopping 2 cups' worth. It will keep your hands and mouth busy, preventing you from turning to other, more-fattening fare. To make it, coat a saucepan with olive oil cooking spray and heat over low to medium heat. Add ½ cup chopped white or yellow onion. Sauté 3 to 4 minutes, or until translucent. Remove from the heat. In a bowl, mix the onion with ½ cup fat-free sour cream, ⅛ teaspoon each of onion powder and black pepper, and 1 teaspoon light canola oil mayonnaise. Use it as a dip for 10 baby carrots, 1 sliced green or red bell pepper, or 2 cups of your favorite raw vegetable.

The Stressed Slender's Top Three Moves

Muscle tension tends to create emotional tension. The following stretches will help to soothe away muscle tension, in turn calming your mind. Try them whenever you feel tense throughout the day. In the morning, look to them to help you start the day focused and relaxed. At night, they'll help you to unwind for bed.

CHILD'S POSE

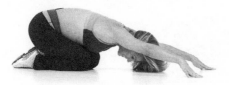

Sit on your heels with your shins against the floor, your big toes touching, your heels relaxed apart, and your knees splayed apart. Bend forward, bringing your tummy into the space between your knees and your forehead onto the floor. Reach your hands either out in front, as shown, or rest them by your feet (whichever is more comfortable and relaxing for you). Inhale deeply, feeling your tummy expand into your thighs and your lower back round. Exhale and feel your body relax. Take 5 deep breaths in this way, imagining that all of your tension is falling out of your forehead and onto the floor. Then move on to the next stretch.

SEATED SIDE STRETCH

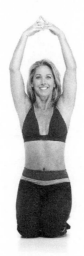

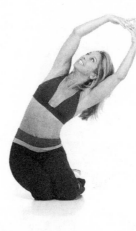

A

Sit on your heels with your shins against the floor, your big toes touching, heels apart, and your knees fairly close together. Lift your arms overhead, clasping your hands together.

B

Exhale as you reach up and over to the left with your fingertips as you simultaneously jut your hips to the right and down. Hold for 3 deep, slow breaths, release, and repeat on the other side.

LEGS UP THE WALL

Inverted yoga postures reverse the action of gravity on the body. When you do a shoulder stand, handstand, or headstand, gravity pulls blood and other fluids toward your head instead of your feet. This upside-down shift also can change your mood, giving you a new perspective on life. Children know this instinctively, which is why you see so many of them placing their heads on the floor! As we grow older, we often forget the deliciously relaxing benefits of going upside down.

The true shoulder stand in yoga, however, can be quite challenging, which is why I recommend this beginning version, called legs up the wall.

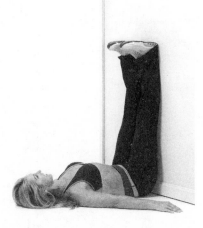

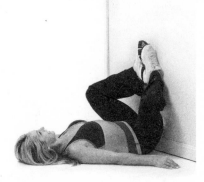

A

B

Sit with one side of your body to a wall. Lower your back onto the floor and shimmy your legs up the wall so your torso forms a right angle with your legs. Allow your legs to completely relax, with your knees soft. Rest your arms and hands at your sides. Hold the position for 1 to 2 minutes.

You can keep your legs extended, as shown at left; bring them into a butterfly position, as shown above; or open them into a V shape. Place them in whatever position is most relaxing for you!

8 THE AFTER BABY TYPE

Yes, You Can Firm Up Your Tummy—
No Matter How Many Babies You've Had!

Most women—even women with washboard abs before pregnancy—tell me that their tummies just are not the same after pregnancy. I've battled this phenomenon myself after the birth of each of my daughters, so I can speak from personal experience!

I had to get in a leotard and appear on television just 6 weeks after giving birth to each of my daughters. Talk about pressure to get back in shape! Although my tummy certainly was not rock hard, I managed to get it presentable within this short period of time. My tummy was still soft and my waistline thick, and I remember feeling as if it would never look the same. Within 6 months of having my first daughter and 9 months after my second, however, I had whittled my waistline down from its widest during pregnancy, 44 inches, to my usual 26 inches. So I'm living proof that it can be done!

To get back in shape, you have to focus on two goals. First, you must lose any excess fat you gained over the course of your pregnancy. Physicians recommend you gain 25 to 35 pounds during pregnancy. The baby, placenta, and extra fluid weigh *at the most* 15 to 20 pounds, so most women are carrying an extra 5 or more pounds after pregnancy than before. Make it your goal to lose most of this extra fat within 6 months of giving birth, as statistics show this is the best weight-loss window for new moms. Women who do not shed the weight during the first 6 months after giving birth tend to still carry that extra weight 10 to 20 years later!

Second, you need to firm up your pelvic floor and abdomen. During your pregnancy, your growing baby stretched and weakened your abdominal muscles. Your pelvic floor muscles—which support your abdomen—are also very weak from the delivery of your baby, so you need to strengthen that area of the body as well.

The tummy-specific movements in the Core Complete routines in Chapter 11 will help you firm all of these body areas, but, depending on your level of fitness, you may not be ready for those routines just yet. If you exercised throughout your pregnancy, you may be able to tackle the tummy-specific exercises as long as you are 6 weeks postpartum. If you were sedentary, you can still achieve good results, but you may need to start with gentler movements, such as the ones described in the "A Test Before You Start" section in Chapter 11, as well as the ones shown in this chapter.

No matter where you start, go easy on yourself! Tackling too much exercise too soon can actually weaken your abdomen, so listen to your body and try not to overdo it. Don't do any jumping or bouncing movements during the first 6 months after pregnancy, as the hormone that helped expand your cervix for the birth of your baby is still present in your body and may increase your risk of a joint injury.

If you're a brand-new mom just out of the hospital, I want you to rest and get to know your baby! Don't attempt to strengthen your abdomen (with the exception of Kegels, deep breathing, walking, and the exercises in "A Test Before You Start" until you have your doctor's approval. Some of the puffiness and looseness you see in your tummy will naturally subside over time as your uterus returns to its prepregnancy size.

TONE YOUR AFTER BABY TUMMY

While everyone will get great results using the Core Diet and Core Moves (which start on page 83 and page 95, respectively), an After Baby Tummy Type can get even more impressive results by focusing on these key strategies, developed to tap into and make the most of her particular biochemistry.

1. Kegels, Kegels, Kegels! Your obstetrician has probably suggested you do Kegel exercises to help build back strength in your pelvic floor. Heed that advice! Kegels not only will help you to strengthen the foundation that supports your abdomen but also will prevent or minimize postpartum problems such as incontinence and low libido. To do one, firm the muscles around your genitals—including your vagina, anus, and urethra—by lifting up and in, as if you were trying to stop yourself from passing wind or leaking urine. As you do this, try not to tighten your tummy, squeeze your legs together, firm your buns, or hold your breath. Hold as long as you can, building up to a maximum of 10 seconds. Then release, rest for 4 seconds, and repeat up to 10 times. Do this several times a day. To help yourself to remember to do them, try doing Kegels whenever you nurse or bottle-feed your baby.

2. Walk as often as possible. Many infants love being pushed in a stroller. As you walk, keep your tummy as firm as possible by zipping up those abs and standing tall with good posture. You can walk soon after giving birth, as long as you listen to your body and stop once you feel fatigued.

3. Practice deep abdominal breathing. Deep breathing will help you to pull in those slack tummy muscles, shortening them to their prepregnancy length. Sit with your back against a wall (for comfort) and your legs crossed. (If you'd like, hold your baby in your lap.) Place one or both hands on your abdomen and notice your breathing. As you inhale, try to expand your tummy into your hand, feeling your tummy come forward, your ribs expand outward, and your chest and collarbones upward. As you exhale, pull everything inward, scooping your tummy inward as much as possible. Hold up to a count of 5. Then repeat 3 to 5 times. Do this several times a day.

4. Modify your crunch technique. Modify the crunching exercises in the Core Complete and the Core Cardio Blast routines in Chapter 11 by bending your knees and pressing them together. This will activate your pelvic floor muscles and help protect your back. Do the plank and reverse crunches with a towel or small ball between your thighs to further activate these muscles and encourage proper technique. To help you remember to do this for the right exercises, I've included notations throughout the exercise routine.

5. Breastfeed rather than formula-feed your baby, if possible, for a year or longer. Breastfeeding expends about 500 calories a day and may help you lose weight. That said, breastfeeding is not a foolproof weight-loss method. Some women drop pounds fast while nursing. Others find their bodies cling to fat until they are done nursing. This may be especially true for women who are older than 35 or who gained more than 35 pounds during pregnancy. I breastfed my first daughter, Kelly, for 9 months and my second daughter, Katie, for 6 months. Just do the best you can.

The After Baby's Top Tummy-Slimming Snack

The nuts and wheat germ in these Mama's Little Helper Brownies give this treat healthful nutrition to boost a busy mom's energy. They also contain calcium, which is so important during nursing. And what snack could be better to satisfy that midafternoon chocolate craving?

Makes 12 brownies

1	package (6 ounces) semisweet (or dark) chocolate chips
3	tablespoons butter
3/4	cup quick-cooking oats
1/3	cup wheat germ toasted, no sugar added
1/3	cup fat-free dry milk
1/2	tablespoon baking powder
1	cup walnuts, chopped
4	egg whites
1/2	cup brown sugar, packed
1	teaspoon vanilla

In a microwave-safe dish, melt the chocolate chips and butter at 80 percent power. (It takes about 45 seconds, depending on the microwave.) Blend well and set aside. In a bowl, combine the oats, wheat germ, dry milk, baking powder, and walnuts. In a large bowl, beat the egg whites with the sugar and vanilla until slightly thick. Stir in the chocolate mixture and then the dry ingredients. Spread in an 8" × 8" × 2" baking dish coated with cooking spray. Bake 20 to 35 minutes at 350°F, until the edges are firm and the top is crisp. Cool completely before cutting or refrigerate overnight before serving.

The After Baby's Top Three Moves

The following movements will help to gently firm your tummy and pelvic floor. Check with your physician before trying these and other exercises described in this book. All moms and deliveries are different. Restrictions may apply to you that prevent your doing these exercises immediately. Begin only after your doctor clears you to exercise, which is usually at least 6 weeks after delivery (or longer if you had a C-section). Once you have the

I TONED MY TUMMY!

KRISTA PHILLIPS

TUMMY TYPE: **After Baby**

AGE: **40**

HOMETOWN: **Grass Valley, California**

RESULTS: **Lost 9½ pounds and 3½ inches from the tummy area in 4 weeks**

LIFE-CHANGING EXPERIENCE: **Can now keep up with her six children**

My husband, Darren, and I started the Tone Your Tummy Type program together because we have six children—the youngest being only 15 months old—and we want to keep up with them far into the future. One day when I was playing with my kids, my knees and ankles ached, and I knew I had to do something. Darren and I decided to change our ways to set a good example for our children.

My weight gain happened slowly over the years. I had my first two children in my early twenties, and the weight came off fairly easily after those pregnancies. Then I had four more children in my thirties and didn't lose the "baby weight" in between. The older I got, the harder it became for me to lose the pounds. Before I knew it, I was 50 pounds overweight.

Prior to starting Denise's program, I felt like a middle-aged slob. I was embarrassed and paranoid. When my husband and I were eating with friends, I felt like everyone was watching me to see if I was eating more than I imagined they thought I should have been eating. I used to feel like saying, "Really, I'm not this fat. I'm really slim—I just have this stuff on the outside of me."

I also started to realize how ridiculous it was that I couldn't keep up with my own children. I was wasting my time being fat. Plus, it was no fun having a big tummy!

okay to exercise, do these moves as often as every day. I recommend you do them first thing in the morning. As a new mom, you're going to be juggling many new responsibilities. Doing your ab work in the morning helps to ensure you get it accomplished and frees you up to focus on your new baby.

You can do the following moves with or without shoes. For your comfort, I recommend you do them on a mat or on carpeting.

Denise's Tone Your Tummy Type program has helped me in several ways. Most important, it has given me the inspiration, knowledge, and tools that I needed to change my eating habits, as well as an exercise routine to shrink my tummy. I need a plan that tells me, "Eat this, exercise this way for this long, and do this routine on this particular day." It has to be spelled out for me, and with this program, it clearly is! The Tone Your Tummy Type program has also helped me learn that I was eating *way* too much. I have discovered that I can be satisfied with a lot less food.

In terms of the exercises, I love the way the routine is broken up. I never get bored. The daily routines are fast-paced, and they aren't ever repetitive.

The recipes are very tasty, easy to prepare, and include unique ingredients I never would have thought of using before. I feed the kids the same foods Darren and I eat most of the time, and they love the food, too!

The best part is, I have so much more energy now—it is truly unbelievable! I actually look forward to the exercise. I wake up earlier in the morning, and I don't feel sluggish in the middle of the day. *Everyone* has been commenting on how I look. It's funny—I weighed about 10 pounds less a year ago, but people say they've never seen me look this slim! The exercise and meal plan have made such a difference in my body that the pounds don't mean nearly as much to me as they used to. My kids have also said I feel thinner when they hug me.

Personally, I can see the bulk of the weight loss in my tummy, but I also see a huge difference in my upper legs. Darren says my back flab is disappearing as well, and I've only just begun!

Thanks to the Tone Your Tummy Type program, I feel so much more hopeful. I now know that I'm not stuck in this fat, blobby body! I have the power to make it disappear.

SIT BACKS

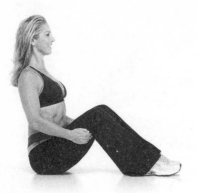

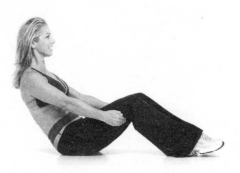

A

Sit with your knees bent and feet on the floor. Press your knees together. Place your hands against your thighs for support.

B

Exhale and round your back, contract your ab muscles, and scoop your tummy inward as you lean back. Rise and repeat for a total of 5 times.

LEG SLIDE

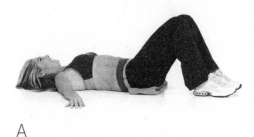

A

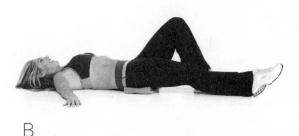

B

While lying on your back with your knees bent, tilt your pelvis backward as you tighten your abs and exhale. Place a small towel under your buttocks. This will help you to tilt your pelvis in the right direction, bringing your lower back toward the floor. Try to bring your belly button to your backbone as you push your lower back into the towel. Place your arms at your sides.

Keeping your spine and hips stable, slide your right heel away from your body as you slowly straighten your right leg. Only go as far as you can keep your back flat. Once you start to feel your back rise, bring your heel back in. Then repeat with the other leg. Complete 3 to 5 leg slides with each leg. You can progress by doing it without the towel and still keeping your lower back flat.

CAT AND COW

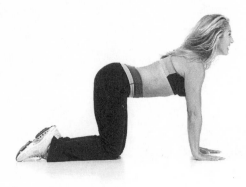

A

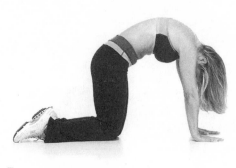

B

Kneel with your palms under your shoulders and your knees under your hips. Inhale.

Exhale as you draw your abdominals in toward your spine and tuck your tailbone, bringing your tailbone and sternum down in an arc. Use your abdominal muscles to do all the work. Inhale and relax. Do 5 repetitions.

9 THE GUY TYPE

The Elusive Six-Pack Is within Your Grasp

A lot of guys remember me from when I was on ESPN for more than 10 years, from 1987 to 1998. Many guys really liked my "Rock-Hard Abs" segments. In honor of them, I thought I would dedicate a chapter just to you guys! Plus, I know that many of my female fans use the advice I offer in my books to help their guys shape up and slim down. So no matter whether you bought this book on your own or your girlfriend or wife has suggested you read this chapter, I welcome you!

The Core Diet plan and the Core Moves exercises described throughout this book will help you to flatten your tummy. If you are chasing after that elusive six-pack that so many men seek, however, you'll need a few extra tactics.

As a man, you have higher levels of the sex hormone testosterone than women do, which makes you more likely to gain fat in your abdomen, compared with other parts of your body. Also, this hormone directs more of your fat to the deepest part of the tummy, where it is most dangerous to your health.

Shedding this tummy fat isn't straightforward. Unlike for women, the answer is *not* lower testosterone levels. In fact, studies show that men with reduced levels of testosterone—through a complicated chain of events—actually accumulate *more* tummy fat than men with higher levels. You need testosterone to build muscle. You also need it for the proper function of the hormone insulin. So, even though this hormone is responsible for your tummy type, trying to influence its levels isn't the answer.

On the other hand, the type of tummy fat most common in men is easier to lose than the tummy fat most women carry around. In fact, you need only a modest amount of exercise to turn things around. A study of 300 men published in *Medicine and Science in Sports and Exercise* found that men with higher levels of cardiorespiratory fitness—levels achieved with roughly 30 daily minutes of exercise—had narrower waist circumferences than men with lower fitness levels. Men considered to have low cardiorespiratory fitness had higher levels of both visceral fat and subcutaneous fat.

TONE YOUR GUY TUMMY

While everyone will get great results using the Core Diet and Core Moves (which start on page 83 and page 95, respectively), a Guy Tummy Type can get even more impressive results by focusing on these key strategies, developed to tap into and make the most of his particular biochemistry.

TOP TUMMY TACTIC | **1. Lift more weights and scale back on the cardio.** If you do a lot of endurance exercise such as running or cycling and hardly any weight training, you'll want to tweak your routine to bring things into a better balance. When it comes to the Guy Tummy Type, some cardio is good, but more weight training is better. Let's face it. We all have only a certain amount of time to put into working out. If you skimp on the weights in order to fit in more running, you need to change your perspective. Cardio burns calories *as you exercise.* Weight training also burns calories during a workout (to a lesser extent than cardio)—but then it burns calories after your workout, as your body busily works to repair and strengthen your muscles. More important, for every pound of muscle you build, you permanently speed your metabolism by up to 50 daily calories. So change your focus and try to fit in your cardio around your weight sessions, making sure to strengthen

I TONED MY TUMMY!

DARREN PHILLIPS

TUMMY TYPE: **Guy**

AGE: **42**

HOMETOWN: **Grass Valley, California**

RESULTS: **Lost 14 pounds and 5 inches from his tummy area in 4 weeks**

LIFE-CHANGING EXPERIENCE: **Got over being embarrassed about his male tummy**

Before I started Denise Austin's Tone Your Tummy Type program, I never took my shirt off in public. I was afraid people wouldn't respect me because I was overweight, and I was particularly self-conscious about my "male tummy" because of my job. As a professional ER nurse, I feel that other people's perceptions of me are important. Who was I to tell someone he should improve his lifestyle when I was a walking candidate for heart disease and diabetes myself? Plus, my father has a history of cardiac problems, and I am a borderline type 2 diabetic, and I'd like to be around to see my six children grow up. So when my wife, Krista, decided to participate in the Tone Your Tummy Type trial, I wholeheartedly joined her.

Except for a few years in high school, I always struggled with tummy fat . . . and my wife's previous daily batch of chocolate chip cookies (the best in the world!) certainly didn't help. As I got older, I ate increasingly more at a sitting to stay satisfied, and I ate the wrong foods. All this, combined with a lack of exercise, led to a stubborn male tummy.

I am so happy I decided to try Denise Austin's Tone Your Tummy Type program because, honestly, this is the first time in my life that I have successfully lost weight. The program has taught me numerous lifestyle skills that have helped me shed an initial 14 pounds. I now eat smaller meals four times a day instead of larger ones two or three times a day. I have also learned that I don't have to eat bread, fat, and meat to feel full. I eat so much less food, but I still feel just as satisfied. The recipes taste great, and I particularly love the freedom I have to eat at my favorite Mexican restaurant!

I have also discovered how much of a difference even moderate exercise has made in the shape of my body and my energy level. Unfortunately, I broke my foot halfway through the program and couldn't perform most of the exercises in phase 2; I know that if that wouldn't have happened, I would have lost twice as much weight by this point. As soon as my foot heals, I'm going to continue to do the exercises exactly as they are written.

Today, instead of feeling self-conscious about my weight, I feel proud—people are telling me how good I look and to keep it up. It feels so great. The Tone Your Tummy Type program is not a weight-loss gimmick—it is an outline for a healthy lifestyle. My wife and I are both so thankful that we've had the opportunity to participate in the program—it has changed our lives!

your major muscle groups no less than three times a week. Both cardio and weights are important for men, so if you're short on time, focus on the weights and scale back on the cardio. (But you do need both—it's a balance.)

2. Cut back on alcohol. Too much alcohol of any kind does in fact create a beer belly. Binge drinking, research shows, is especially problematic. In one study that compared types of drinks and frequency of drinking on abdominal fat, researchers determined that people who consumed more than three to four beverages per drinking episode—even if those episodes were infrequent—had more abdominal fat than people who consumed small amounts of alcohol regularly. The bottom line: One beer a night is better than four beers on a Friday after work.

3. Replace saturated fat with polyunsaturated fat. I know you guys like a good burger—really, who doesn't?—but consider an occasional switch to the veggie variety. The Core Diet outlined in this book will help you trade saturated fats with healthier polyunsaturated fats. Saturated fat found in fatty animal products (full-fat milk, fatty cuts of meat) tends to accumulate deep in the abdomen, whereas polyunsaturated fats (in sunflower, corn, and soybean oils as well as fish) do not tend to cause tummy weight gain.

The Guy's Top Tummy-Slimming Snack

Try the following Protein-Packed Smoothie after your workouts to help your muscles recover. In a blender, combine 1 tablespoon wheat germ, 1 cup fat-free milk, 3 ounces tofu with calcium sulfate, 1 cup blackberries (for a really thick, frosty smoothie, don't thaw berries if using frozen ones), and ½ teaspoon almond or vanilla extract. Blend until smooth.

The Guy's Top Three Moves

To sculpt that six-pack, you need to challenge those ab muscles in new ways. The following moves will do just that. I recommend you roll out of bed and do them right away each morning, in addition to the other routines outlined in Chapter 11. Research shows you're more likely to stick with an exercise program when you do it first thing. These ab exercises focus right where you need it: the transverse abdominis, obliques, and the rectus abdominis. Your core muscles *will* get fit!

LOW HOVER I

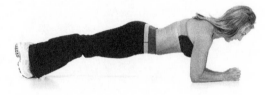

A

Kneel on your hands and knees. Extend your legs and bend your arms, so your body weight is supported on your forearms and the balls of your feet, as shown. Hold for 30 seconds.

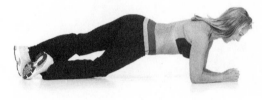

B

After holding for 30 seconds, bend your right knee, bringing it down and to the left in a twisting motion. You should not feel the effort in your obliques, the love handles area of the abdomen. Alternate bending and twisting with your right and left knees for 30 seconds.

ROPE CLIMB

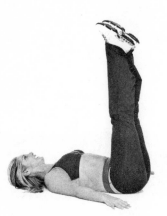

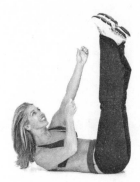

A

Lie on your back. Lift your legs and extend them toward the ceiling. Rest your arms at your sides, palms facing down.

B

Lift your arms toward the ceiling and grab onto your imaginary rope. Lift your head, neck, and upper back. Now climb your rope, reaching up with your left hand, as shown, and then reaching up with your right. Continue alternating sides for 1 minute.

OBLIQUES FIRMER
(OR BICYCLE)

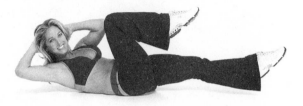

The bicycle is among the most effective
abdominal exercises ever invented. Lie on
your back with your knees bent and your
feet lifted off the floor. Place your fingertips
behind your head and your elbows out to the
sides. Firm your tummy as you lift your
head, neck, and shoulders. Keep your
elbows straight out from your ears—you
should not be able to see your elbows! Bring
your left elbow and right knee toward each
other as you extend your left leg. Then
switch, bringing your right leg and left elbow
toward one another. Continue to pedal your
imaginary bicycle in this way for 1 minute.

PART THREE

THE TUMMY TYPE ESSENTIALS

10 THE CORE DIET

The Eating Plan That Turns Down Inflammation and Turns Up Your Body's Ability to Burn Fat

Now that you've discovered your tummy type and your individual strategies for slimming your midsection, you're ready to learn about my Core Diet. In this chapter you will learn which foods and beverages contribute to tummy fat and which ones help you shed it.

All tummy types follow the same eating plan. The eating strategies in this chapter effectively whittle away tummy fat—no matter your tummy type. The meal plan you will use for the next 4 weeks (2 weeks for phase 1 and 2 weeks for phase 2) includes optimal amounts of important tummy-slimming nutrients such as fiber (to stabilize blood sugar and reduce hunger and inflammation), omega-3 fatty acids from fish and other sources (to improve metabolism and reduce inflammation), fruits and vegetables (to reduce inflammation), and calcium (to encourage the burning of abdominal fat). It also minimizes tummy-fattening nutrients such as refined carbohydrates, added sugars, and saturated fats, all of which turn up inflammation and encourage tummy fat storage.

In Chapter 15, you'll find dozens of quick, easy, and delicious recipes that help you to effortlessly maximize these tummy-slimming foods while minimizing tummy-fattening foods. These recipes will help you to quickly make the shift to Tone Your Tummy Type eating.

In Chapter 12, you'll find my 2-week Jump-Start Phase menus that will take you one day at a time through the first 14 days of the Core Diet. This meal plan mixes and matches the recipes from Chapter 15, organizing them into 1,300-calorie daily menus for quick fat loss. In this rapid weight-loss phase of the plan, you can expect to lose up to 5 pounds a week. You will see and feel results in just 2 weeks! This is the jump-start meal plan I personally follow when I need to shape up and slim down when filming my television show and DVD or right before an important photo shoot. It's that fast and effective! Just think—in 2 weeks you could be 10 pounds lighter than you are right now! That's certainly motivating to me!

In Chapter 13, you'll find the second phase of the Core Diet—what I call my 2-week Keep-On-Losing Phase. This meal plan builds on your initial success, allowing you to consume 1,500 calories a day. Because you'll be eating more than you were in the first 2 weeks of the program, the 2-week Keep-On-Losing Phase may feel like a culinary indulgence! But, rest assured, you will continue to lose weight. Although I've included meal plans that span 2 weeks, you can remain in the Keep-On-Losing Phase for as long as it takes to reach your goal. (In Chapter 14, you'll find advice for varying your diet and keeping things interesting and fun on the way to your goal.)

THE ELEMENTS OF TONE YOUR TUMMY TYPE EATING

How does the Core Diet help you to shed tummy fat? The menus and recipes emphasize key nutrients (nutrients you will learn more about in the section "Tummy-Taming Ingredients," below) that work together to shrink tummy fat, reduce inflammation throughout your body, stabilize insulin levels, turn down hunger, and boost energy. At the same time, they minimize foods and nutrients known to contribute to tummy fat. (You'll learn more about these nutrients under the heading "Tummy-Troubling Foods on page 88.")

On each phase of the plan, you'll fill your body with what it needs to burn fat—and none of the ingredients that tend to hinder fat burning. Each day you'll eat balanced meals, consuming about 50 percent of your calories from carbohydrate (to fuel your workouts), 20 to 25 percent from healthful fats (mostly from unsaturated fats to raise your good HDL cholesterol and turn down hunger), and 25 to 30 percent from lean protein (to help your muscles repair after your workout, stabilize your blood sugar, and keep you satisfied between meals).

On each day of the plan, I've made sure that your meals and snacks are evenly balanced to stabilize blood sugar levels and minimize hunger. You'll find that your snacks provide true staying power and allow you to lose weight without feeling deprived.

Tummy-Taming Ingredients

Each day of your meal plan includes a number of health-promoting ingredients that work together to help you burn tummy fat fast. These ingredients include:

Fiber. Each day of the plan includes an abundance of fruits, vegetables, legumes, and whole grains, all of which provide nearly 30 daily grams of fiber. A number of studies have linked diets high in fiber with lower indicators of inflammation. For example, in one study published in the *American Journal of Clinical Nutrition*, researchers tracked the diets, exercise habits, and levels of C-reactive protein (a blood component that's a measure of inflammation throughout the body) of 524 adults for more than a year. The more fiber each participant consumed, the lower their blood levels of C-reactive protein. A separate study published in *Diabetes Care* yielded similar results, linking the consumption of bran and other whole grains to reduced markers of inflammation in 902 women with diabetes.

In addition to reducing inflammation—which in turn may reduce tummy fat—dietary fiber can stabilize insulin levels, which reduces hunger and allows you to feel satisfied on fewer calories. These reduced insulin levels will also help to contribute to a slimmer midsection.

Omega-3 fatty acids. In Chapter 1, I mentioned the importance of fish oil supplements. These supplements are a rich source of omega-3 fatty acids. Few people consume enough of this important fat, which may help you shed tummy fat in two important ways. First, consumption of these fats has been linked to an increased presence and action of fat-burning enzymes. In short, they encourage your body to waste energy—in the form of stored belly fat—as heat. Second, omega-3 fatty acids help calm inflammation throughout the body, which also may enable you to shed fat faster.

Although some experts recommend you eat fish as often as possible in order to cash in on these wonderful benefits, I'm not quite as gung ho. In addition to the wonderful tummy-slimming omega-3 fatty acids, many varieties of ocean-caught fish contain many different contaminants, including mercury and PCBs. (Fish oil supplements, on the other hand, have been purified and do not contain these harmful contaminants.) For that reason, you will find a variety of omega-3 fatty acid sources on the meal plan, including fish (from varieties that are generally lower in mercury), flax, olive oil, canola oil, walnuts, and sunflower seeds and oil. Roughly one-quarter of the meals you will eat on this plan are rich in omega-3s.

Fruits and vegetables. Scientists have known for many years that fruits and vegetables are nature's power foods when it comes to good health. They house many nutrients that help prevent cancer, heart disease, and diabetes and reduce inflammation. On this plan, you'll eat an average of six servings of fruits and vegetables every day.

Calcium. The Tone Your Tummy Type program includes 1,000 daily milligrams of calcium in the form of low-fat dairy products such as yogurt. This will do more than simply strengthen your bones, as a growing number of studies show that this mineral may help you to burn tummy fat. Stored inside of fat cells, calcium plays a crucial role in regulating how the body stores and breaks down fat. In one study, researchers from Purdue University in West Lafayette, Indiana, found that a high-calcium diet increased fat burning following a meal. In another study, researchers determined that obese adults who ate three servings of fat-free yogurt a day lost 22 percent more weight and 61 percent more body fat than participants who cut calories but did not eat yogurt. Most important, the yogurt eaters *lost 81 percent more tummy fat* than non–yogurt eaters.

For best results, get your calcium from food rather than supplements, as research shows consumption of dairy products—particularly yogurt—is more effective at burning tummy fat than taking calcium supplements. No one knows precisely why, but some other component present in dairy products may enable the body to absorb or use calcium.

So there you have it. Fiber, omega-3 fats, fruits and vegetables, and the right dairy products are the magical ingredients that make the Tone Your Tummy Type program work. As a side note, these foods are also cornerstones of the traditional Mediterranean style diet. A study that compared this diet to the more prudent American Heart Association diet, which restricts all fats (including omega-3 fats), found that participants on the Mediterranean diet lost more weight than participants on the American Heart Association diet, even though they ate the same number of calories! Also, the Mediterranean diet participants significantly reduced markers of inflammation and improved insulin levels.

TOP 10 TUMMY-SLIMMING SUPERFOODS

You'll find the following 10 Tone Your Tummy Type superfoods often in your meal plan and recipes. They all include the important tummy-slimming ingredients mentioned in this chapter.

PORTION OF FOOD	TUMMY-TONING ASSETS
Fish, 3 oz cooked, no fat added (120–175 calories)	Rich in omega-3 fats
Walnuts, 1 oz (185 calories, 2 g fiber)	Rich in omega-3 fats and fiber
Almonds, 1 oz (170 calories, 3 g fiber)	Rich in omega-3 fats and a little calcium and fiber
Broccoli, 1 cup raw, 1/2 cup cooked (30 calories, 2 g fiber)	Low-calorie food with a little calcium and fiber
Spinach, 1/2 cup cooked or 1 cup raw (10–20 calories; 2 g fiber)	Low-calorie food with a little calcium and fiber
Extra-virgin olive oil, 1 tsp (40 calories)	Rich in omega-3 fats
Soy cheese, 1 slice (40 calories)	Little to no saturated fat and a good dose of calcium Low-calorie food
Fat-free ricotta cheese, 1/4 cup (40 calories)	No saturated fat and a good dose of calcium Low-calorie food
Fat-free milk, 1 cup (83 calories)	No saturated fat and a good dose of calcium Low-calorie food
Fat-free plain yogurt, 6 oz (80 calories)	No saturated fat and a good dose of calcium Low-calorie food

Tummy-Troubling Foods

So, now that you know what you will be eating over the next few weeks, it's important to understand what you *won't* be eating and why. The Tone Your Tummy Type program minimizes refined carbohydrates, added sugars, saturated fat, and trans fat, all of which increase inflammation and contribute to abdominal fat.

Refined carbohydrates and added sugars. Although the Tone Your Tummy Type program is not a low-carbohydrate diet, the plan does restrict certain types of carbohydrates. The majority of the carbs you will eat come in the form of fruits, vegetables, legumes, and whole grains. This plan includes very little added sugar or refined carbohydrates in the form of snack crackers, white bread, and pasta. Added sugars and refined foods made from white flour tend to raise blood sugar and insulin levels, triggering hunger and abdominal fat storage. These foods also increase inflammation throughout the body.

Saturated fats. Saturated fat comes from meat, dairy, and other animal products. On

DENISE'S RULES FOR HEALTHY CHOICES AT THE DELI COUNTER

Deli meats often contain unnecessary sodium, nitrates, and fat. To make smart choices at the deli counter, ask to see the nutrition facts label for any type of deli meat you wish to purchase, and then use these guidelines to decide whether to buy or pass.

☐ Do not buy bologna, sausage, salami, bacon, pepperoni, hot dogs, and pastrami made from fatty beef or pork. These meats are high in fat and sodium. Look for healthier, leaner versions of these products made from turkey or chicken breast. Make sure the cured products that you buy contain no more than 3 grams of fat, 1 gram of saturated fat, and 300 milligrams of sodium per ounce.

☐ Choose reduced-fat and reduced-sodium cheeses. These cheeses generally contain 25 percent less fat and sodium than regular cheese but offer the same taste and consistency.

☐ Make sure any cheese contains *no more* than 6 grams of fat, 4 grams of saturated fat, and 200 milligrams of sodium per ounce.

☐ Make sure meat contains *no more* than 3 grams of fat, 1 gram of saturated fat, and 300 milligrams of sodium per ounce.

☐ Choose organic meats and cheese whenever possible to avoid antibiotics, artificial colorings, and preservatives. Organic farming also generally results in more humane treatment of the livestock.

this plan, all of your animal protein sources are lean, minimizing saturated fat as much as possible. You'll consume low-fat dairy products, skinless chicken breasts, fish, and other sources of lean protein. Various studies have linked diets high in saturated fat with high levels of C-reactive protein. Also, diets high in saturated fat tend to spike insulin levels, triggering hunger and abdominal fat storage.

Trans fats. These synthetic fats also increase inflammation throughout the body. Trans fats extend the shelf life of food, which is why you'll find them in many foods that are sold in a box or bag. Typically found in cookies, candy, crackers, margarine, and baked goods, trans fats are particularly troublesome because they not only raise total cholesterol and LDL levels—they can lower HDL levels, too. This makes them even more dangerous than saturated fats.

Since the government began requiring food companies to list trans fats on their food labels, more and more "trans-free" products have been hitting the supermarket shelves. Don't, however, be tricked into believing that "trans-free!" automatically means healthy. Fats lend a certain mouthfeel to foods—a particular creaminess to candies, margarine, and other treats and a crispiness to crackers and cookies. It's hard, but not impossible, for the manufacturer to eliminate the trans fats and maintain this creaminess and crispiness.

So check your label before deeming your trans-free food as healthy. Although some of these products are true blessings, others are really wolves in sheep's clothing. In some products, you may find that the manufacturer has replaced trans fats with another unhealthful fat. Steer clear of ingredients high in saturated fat such as coconut or palm oil (often called tropical oils) or stearic acid–rich vegetable oil, sometimes listed as inter-esterified vegetable oil.

A FEW WORDS ABOUT YOUR TUMMY ON ALCOHOL

During phases 1 and 2 of the Tone Your Tummy Type program, I recommend you refrain as much as possible from drinking, which is why I do not include any alcohol in your meal plan. Although alcohol is not necessarily a tummy-troubling food, many studies show that it tends to cause your resolve to unravel. After a glass of beer, the cheese curls and potato chips look crunchier, the nuts saltier, and the cheese yummier. Alcohol simply tends to induce the type of mindless eating that you can't afford to slip into while you are trying to lose weight.

Once you reach your weight-loss goal, you may include up to one drink a day if you desire, as long as you do so with or after a meal and never on an empty stomach! This type of moderate drinking may help you maintain your weight loss, as some research shows that a moderate intake of alcohol helps reduce your risk for inflammation. In one study, participants who consumed one to seven alcoholic beverages a week tended to have lower blood levels of several inflammatory markers than those who did not drink. Five ounces

I TONED MY TUMMY!

DARLENE GLASSMEYER
TUMMY TYPE: **After Baby**
AGE: **34**
HOMETOWN: **Westland, Michigan**
RESULTS: **Lost 8 pounds and 5 inches around her tummy in 4 weeks**
LIFE-CHANGING EXPERIENCE: **Became a positive role model for her two girls**

These days, kids are bombarded with conflicting images. They see stick-thin models in magazines and on TV but then numerous overweight people walking the streets. Of course I wanted to lose my tummy to improve my health and appearance, but, more important, I wanted to be a positive role model for my daughters. I wanted to show them that being fit means incorporating the right combination of exercise and proper nutrition. I want health and fitness to be as second nature to them as brushing their teeth.

I first started struggling with my weight—particularly, my tummy—after my second pregnancy (my daughter is 6 months old now). The pounds I gained with my second daughter combined with the leftover pounds from my first one just seemed to stick with me no matter what I did. Both my daughters were born via C-section, so it took a while before I was even ready to start trying to get back into shape. I was always pretty slender, so the bulge around my middle didn't sit well with me. I hated "hiding" in big, baggy clothes.

Exercise-wise, I walked and took ballet and jazz classes, but I never got into a set routine. I would do well for a couple of weeks and then get lazy.

I am so happy I decided to join the Tone Your Tummy Type trial. It has really done the trick for me. The food plan includes the right combination of fats, carbohydrates, and protein. These

of wine, 1½ ounces of hard liquor, or 12 ounces of beer supply the dose of alcohol needed to realize this effect for women.

It's important that if you drink, you do so moderately and regularly. If you save up all of your daily drinks for one wild weekend night, you may do much more harm than good, as other research has linked binge drinking with increased amounts of tummy fat.

The American Heart Association warns not to start drinking alcohol if you're a non-drinker, and definitely get permission from your doctor before you decide to have a daily drink, as it may wreak havoc with a medication that you're taking.

nutrients are perfectly balanced every day. Thinking back to my previous diet, I know I had high-carb days and high-calorie days, even if the foods I was eating were healthy. Denise's Tone Your Tummy Type plan does the balancing for me—I don't have to think about whether I'm eating enough of one thing or another.

The recipes in the program are easy to prepare, and the meals fill me up until it's time to eat again. I also no longer snack between lunch and dinner (the afternoon used to be my biggest snacking time).

I also enjoy the exercises on the program, particularly the exercise ball and Pilates moves. Denise is such a great motivator. Sometimes when I feel as if there is no way in the world I can do another rep, she gives me hope!

My favorite part of the plan is the simplicity. I'm busy. I work 40 hours a week. I'm a mom to two girls under the age of 4. I'm a wife. I also help my 74-year-old mother, who has dementia. The plan is easy to follow and fits well into my hectic, stress-filled schedule. I truly believe anyone can do it. It's wonderful to know it was designed by Denise Austin—she really knows her stuff about fitness, nutrition, muscles, and anatomy.

I lost 8 pounds and 5 inches on the Tone Your Tummy Type program, and I'm still going. I dropped a clothing size—a nice surprise! People have noticed my weight loss. My husband says my tummy feels smaller when he hugs me, and my dance instructor commented that my balance is much improved, which is no doubt the result of stronger, leaner abs.

Since I started the Tone Your Tummy Type program, I have so much more energy. I feel great about myself, and my newfound confidence carries over into everything I do. Denise's program is wonderful, and it works—I saw results so fast! And I know my lifestyle is rubbing off on my girls, which is an amazing feeling. Thank you for the opportunity!

FEEDING A BUSY FAMILY WHILE TRIMMING YOUR TUMMY

As a mom, I know that it can be hard to take care of yourself while taking care of your family. If your day is anything like mine, it's a wonder you eat at all. But please hear this: You *deserve* to be healthy! And believe me, it's not that difficult to incorporate certain tummy type eating strategies into your family's menu. Doing so will make life easier and better for all of you. Not only will you be able to stay on your plan, you'll be teaching your family great eating habits, too.

To make sure I (and my girls and husband) not only eat but eat healthfully, I have created some shortcuts to meal prep. On Sunday, I chop boneless, skinless chicken breasts into small pieces, add a little salt and pepper, and stir-fry a whole batch. I store the chicken in single-serving zipper-lock bags in the refrigerator. My mom did this for my four siblings and me while we were growing up, and I saw how much it streamlined our dinner preparation.

My girls play lacrosse, and I never miss their games. To keep all of us on schedule, I must have a meal ready to serve so that we can all eat within 5 minutes and then head off to practice or a game. The precooked chicken allows me to do this. I throw the chicken pieces into fajitas with taco seasoning, stir-fry them with vegetables, top them with barbecue sauce and provolone cheese, or mix them with teriyaki sauce and serve over rice.

I encourage you to follow the Core Diet plan to a T for the first 4 weeks. Once you've reached your goals, try some of my favorite timesaving tips to maintain your Tone Your Tummy Type results and feed your family well, for good!

* I make a big, hearty salad with fresh vegetables, cheese, avocado, beans, and the precooked chicken. My whole family enjoys the salad on the side, and it's a main course for me. I use organic packaged salads because they're so convenient.

* I love homemade soups, but if I don't have time to make them myself, I swing by the grocery store and pick up some homemade soup from the deli. I choose minestrone, lentil, vegetable, black bean, or chicken noodle, and I avoid cream-based or heavy-looking soups. It's the next best thing to making my own soup, and it's a lot quicker and healthier than ordering fast food.

* I make fruit smoothies for my girls in a blender using acai berries (available at health food stores), frozen blueberries, frozen strawberries, half a banana, a splash of orange or apple juice, a few ice cubes, and yogurt. The girls can drink this in the car on the way to school, and I bring along wheat toast spread with a little peanut butter.

* I slice fresh tomatoes and top them with a little olive oil, fresh basil, and mozzarella. It takes just a few minutes and tastes like a gourmet meal.

* I make my own trail mix at home with almonds, raisins, and granola. I like to buy prepared trail mixes, too, but I avoid varieties packed with candy, chocolate, or yogurt-covered fruit and nuts that add unnecessary sugar.

* I like to serve baked potatoes, both Idaho potatoes and sweet potatoes. We top them with vegetables, salsa, cheese, and a little light butter for a quick meal.

* Sometimes I serve sandwiches packed with fresh vegetables for another all-in-one quick meal.

* Thin, organic, boneless, butterflied pork chops are another favorite meal. I mix them with bay leaves, apple cider, salt and pepper, and apricot preserves, and then pan-fry them in a skillet. When they're nearly done, I add fresh sugar snap peas to the pan.

* I like to make my own fried rice, too. I start the skillet with a little olive oil, and I add chopped onions, scallions, frozen baby peas, and a can of carrots. I then add cooked rice (a mixture of brown and jasmine) and two scrambled eggs, and I throw in pieces of the precooked chicken—and that's a complete meal!

* Another favorite is baked ziti. In a large bowl, I mix together fat-free ricotta cheese, fresh parsley, one egg, part-skim shredded mozzarella, 2 cups of prepared spaghetti sauce, and a little garlic powder. I pour it over whole wheat pasta (penne style) in a 13" × 9" baking pan, and I top it with Parmesan cheese, bake, and serve with a green salad.

* I boil eggs once a week and store the hard-cooked eggs in the refrigerator. I slice the eggs in half, scoop out the yolks, and give them to my dog. I refill the whites with a little hummus. It's so tasty! For the kids, I make regular deviled eggs with a little mayonnaise.

READY TO GET COOKING?

So, there you have it: the basics of the Core Diet. Very simple, very livable, very delicious! I've collected all of the inflammation-fighting, fat-blasting Core Diet Recipes into one simple-to-use list in Chapter 15—ready for your mouth to water? You will find tasty and easy-to-throw-together recipes that even the most novice cook or busy mom can pull off. These are the same recipes that I cook up for my family every day. I'm confident that you will love them as much as I do!

11 THE CORE MOVES

Burn Fat Three Times Faster Than Traditional Exercise Plans by Following These Incredibly Efficient Routines

Welcome to my Core Moves fitness plan. This exciting program—based on the latest science of shrinking tummy fat—works for all tummy types. The research is clear: No matter the underlying cause of your tummy fat, you must exercise in order to see real and lasting results.

My Core Moves focus on three essential but often underplayed types of exercise to help you burn tummy fat and trim tummy flab. With this successful fitness system, you will see results in record time. In roughly 20 minutes of formal exercise a day, you'll put your body through all of the paces needed to trim your tummy. You'll wage a three-pronged attack on tummy fat with the following routines.

* 10-Minute Core Complete routine—to shape and trim your midsection
* 20-Minute Core Cardio Blast—to burn fat, sculpt sexy muscle, and boost your metabolism
* 1-Minute Easy Fidgetsizers—to increase circulation and burn calories

The two formal exercise routines—the 10-Minute Core Complete and the 20-Minute Core Cardio Blast—include only the movements you need. They allow you to make extremely efficient use of your time. You spend your day doing 90 million things at once, right? Well, these routines are no different. Rather than isolating various types of exercise—say, by doing power walking in the morning to count toward your cardio, hitting the weight room later in the day to tone your entire body, and doing some crunches at night to sculpt your midsection—the two formal routines in this chapter help you accomplish multiple goals at once.

The 10-Minute Core Complete routine: This routine zeros in on and sculpts the beautiful muscles that line your tummy, waistline, and back—your "core." This routine incorporates the most effective movements *proven in scientific research* to shape, elongate, and firm your entire midsection.

The 20-Minute Core Cardio Blast: This routine features a three-for-one interval-training workout. You'll get your heart rate up with cardio to burn the fat that's hiding that slender waistline of yours. The routine integrates strength training with weights, so you'll build lean, sexy muscle throughout your body to improve your posture (which alone will automatically take an inch off your waistline) and boost your metabolism (which will help you burn more calories all day long, even when you're not moving). I also picked strengthening and cardio movements that focus on your abs—so you'll continue to firm your core in this routine.

The 1-Minute Easy Fidgetsizers: You'll also get in the habit of doing informal activity (the 1-Minute Fidgetsizers) whenever you find yourself waiting (in line, at the doctor's office, in traffic). These simple movements will help you crank up your daily calorie burn and eliminate boredom at the same time. Never again will you feel agitated while waiting. You'll just do a fidgetsizer instead. These 1-minute movements may seem easy and simple—and they are! But they add up over the course of the day. By the end of the day, your fidgetsizers will help you to burn up to 500 additional calories!

It doesn't get any more efficient than this! Let's take a closer look at each of your routines, starting with my 1-Minute Easy Fidgetsizers.

1-MINUTE EASY FIDGETSIZERS

When I was working on this book, I flew from Washington, D.C., to California to film my new DVD, *Boot Camp*. During the 6-hour flight, I noticed a few passengers like myself who were getting up often to move. I don't like sitting still, so during a long flight I find myself walking around, stretching, and just generally fidgeting. I move and twist my body by doing side bends, forward bends, and twists. I also drink lots of bottled water, so I often have to get up to use the bathroom. I believe it helps me to feel great when I arrive at my destination. It both fights fat and prevents jet lag—and it's great for circulation, too!

Turns out, this type of spontaneous movement can burn up to 500 extra calories a day! Researchers at the Mayo Clinic have been studying how unconscious exercise—what I like to call 1-Minute Fidgetsizers—helps people control their weight. Of course, these researchers don't give what they study a name that's as easy to remember and say as "unconscious exercise" or even "fidgeting." They use the more formal and scientific-sounding term *nonexercise activity thermogenesis* (NEAT).

Whether you call it NEAT, 1-Minute Fidgetsizers, or just plain squirminess, these little everyday movements add up to major calorie burn. In a fascinating study published in the highly esteemed journal *Science,* these researchers determined that this type of unconscious fidgeting often makes the difference between being thin and being fat. It's what allows some people to overeat on a regular basis and not gain an ounce.

In this study, the researchers overfed volunteers 1,000 calories every day. Because it takes 3,500 calories to build a pound of fat, this type of overeating should have padded each of the participants with an extra 16 pounds by the conclusion of the 8-week study. Yet weight gain varied tremendously, with some participants gaining only 2 pounds over 8 weeks! The researchers realized that the participants who gained the least amount of weight tended to compensate for the extra calories they were eating by unconsciously moving around. They incessantly tapped their feet, stretched out their backs, and shook their legs.

Right about now you might be wondering whether a habitual sitter can change to become a habitual mover. No researcher has conducted an experiment to answer that question, but my experience tells me that one can. Think of my 1-Minute Fidgetsizers as a habit that you are building over time. The more you try to include them into your day, the more you'll find yourself moving. Make it your goal to do 10 of them a day—for a total of 10 minutes.

You'll find specific fidgetsizers on pages 100 to 104. Do them all for 1 minute each. I love to do the four stretches (side bend, seated twist, seated forward bend, and seated back bend) when I travel. They really help to counteract the tension that can set in when I have no other choice but to sit for long periods of time.

To start, I recommend that you follow this golden rule of fidgetsizing:

Whenever you find yourself waiting—sitting in an airplane, car, or train; seated at the doctor's office; watching your child play sports—find a way to move, even if all you do is tap your feet.

DENISE'S 1-MINUTE FIDGETSIZERS

Try to do at least 10 of the following 1-Minute Fidgetsizers every day.

Denise's energizing standing roll-down and roll-up (page 100)

Side bend (page 101)

Seated twist (page 102)

Seated forward bend (page 103)

Seated back bend (page 104)

Power walk for 1 minute (around the block, through an airport, while talking on the phone, down office hallways)

Climb one to two flights of stairs

Tighten your tummy, release, and tighten again (over and over for 1 minute)

Tighten muscles throughout your body for 1 minute

Check your posture; zip up those abs!

March in place

Stretch and reach for the sky

Do one of your tummy type moves

For example, when waiting for a flight at the airport, I try to power walk the concourses. Whenever I find myself waiting in a line at the grocery store, I do some isometrics. I tighten up various muscles in my body—my arms, my legs, my buns, my abs—for about 5 seconds and then release. I also check my posture, making sure my abs are zipped up, as if I were trying to fit into a pair of tight jeans, and my shoulder blades are down, squeezed together and low on my back.

Periodically, when working at home, I like to take little stretching and strengthening breaks. I often place my palms on the kitchen counter, step back with my feet, and bring my body into a right angle, reaching back through my tailbone as I scoop my abs up and in (like a modified downward dog in yoga).

A few times a day I also reenergize with a standing roll-down and roll-up (shown on page 100). I recently suggested this little movement to one of my neighbors, who took my words of wisdom to heart and began rolling down a few times a day. A few weeks later there was a knock at my door. It was my neighbor Chris, showing me her tummy and explaining how this one simple move had worked wonders! Ever since then I've been calling this little roll-down my "natural tummy tuck."

Every hour on the hour—while on my computer or watching television—I do some type of abdominal strengthening. I might lift my knees to my chest, get on the floor for some crunches, or simply tighten my tummy in an isometric contraction. Whenever I find myself stuck in a seated position for a long period of time, I do the following stretches to help keep me energized, prevent back pain, and—most important—increase the circulation to my tummy and waistline. Here are some of my favorites.

DENISE'S ENERGIZING STANDING ROLL-DOWN AND ROLL-UP

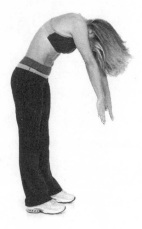

A

Stand with good posture, tuck your chin to your chest, and bend forward, scooping your abs up and in as you bend.

B

Dangle your hands to the floor and imagine someone has placed a belt around your tummy and is pulling it up. Exhale and slowly roll up, keeping your abs scooping upward the entire time. Keep your knees soft, not locked.

The Tummy Type Essentials

SIDE BEND

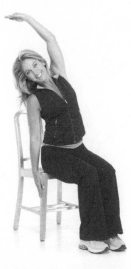

Extend your left arm overhead. Keeping your hips stationary, bend laterally to the right to stretch your left side. Then do the same to the left. I love this stretch, as it helps energize my back, which, now that I'm almost 50, can become stiff when I'm seated for long periods of time.

SEATED TWIST

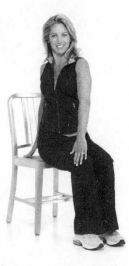

Place your hands on your knees. Sit tall,
reaching your tailbone and sitting bones
down into your seat and the crown of your
head up toward the ceiling. Exhale as you
twist to the right, starting the twist from
your tailbone and moving up your spine as
you revolve your torso. Then face center and
repeat to the other side.

SEATED
FORWARD BEND

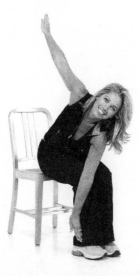

Place your hands on your knees. Sit tall,
reaching your tailbone and sitting bones
down into your seat and the crown of your
head up toward the ceiling. Exhale and bend
forward and to the right, sliding your left
arm down the outside of your right leg and
extending your right arm toward the ceiling.
Hold for 10 to 15 seconds, rise, and repeat
on the other side.

SEATED
BACK BEND

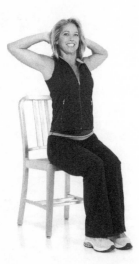

Sit tall, reaching your tailbone and sitting
bones down into your seat and the crown of
your head up toward the ceiling. Pull in your
tummy and place your fingertips behind your
head and elbows out to the sides. Inhale as
you lift up through your breastbone and
back through your elbows, arching slightly
through your upper back and feeling a
stretch in your chest.

HOW THE CORE MOVES SCULPT YOUR TUMMY

You may have heard that you cannot spot-reduce parts of your body through exercise. To some extent that's true. You could do 1,000 crunches every day, and—in the absence of cardio, diet, and allover body toning—you would not experience great results.

So, in that regard, crunches do little to whittle away tummy fat. That's okay, because your other Core Moves routine (the 20-Minute Core Cardio Blast) will take care of that goal. This 10-Minute Core Complete routine can, however, train and sculpt the beautiful and sexy layer of muscle that currently may be hiding underneath your tummy fat. Sculpting these muscles will help to build the lean, firm muscle you need to hold your internal organs in place (preventing them from rounding outward), improve your posture (which lengthens and shrinks the appearance of your midsection), and tighten up the abdominal muscles themselves, which can sag and pooch outward from lack of use, pregnancy, or menopause.

The 10-minute routine strengthens, lengthens, and sculpts the following key tummy areas.

* **The six-pack.** Also known as the upper rectus abdominis, the six-pack section of your tummy starts at your navel and ends at the bottom of your rib cage. Connective tissue that runs through this muscle creates a six-pack appearance in lean, fit people.

* **The lower tummy.** Also called the lower end of the rectus abdominis, this section of the front of the tummy starts at the pubic bone and ends at the navel. Weakness here allows internal organs to pooch out, creating a rounded appearance below the navel, even if you have no noticeable tummy fat.

* **The corset muscle.** Also called the transverse abdominis, this deep muscle lies beneath your six-pack muscle, obscuring it from view. This very important but little used muscle helps you contract your abdomen and draw your tummy inward. When you suck in your tummy to look good in a photo or feel yourself let out a "tummy grunt" during a challenging game of tennis, you are using your transverse muscle. When you tone this muscle, you allow it to do its job—support and lengthen your entire midsection. You can think of it as a natural girdle, as it hugs your internal organs inward.

* **The waistline.** Also known as the internal and external obliques, these abdominal muscles help you side bend, twist, and rotate your torso. Your external obliques sit

closest to the surface toward the front of your waist, with the internal obliques located deeper and closer to your back.

* **The back.** Not a lot of women and men focus on their back muscles when trying to shrink and firm their abdomens—and that's really too bad! Not only does toning your back prevent back pain and improve your posture, it shrinks your love handles as well as any back flab. Many muscles work together to support your back, but one of the more important ones when it comes to the shape of your tummy is called the latissimus dorsi. Located on each side of your spine, this muscle helps you to extend, rotate, and pull your arms toward your body. When you sculpt and tone this muscle, you create a slant from your armpits to your waist, with the muscle fanning inward as it descends down your torso. This consequently makes your waistline appear smaller.

* **The pelvic-floor muscles.** If many people neglect the back when trying to firm up their midsection, even more ignore the pelvic floor. Yet firming this area of the body is essential to creating a healthy, firm, toned midsection. Your pelvic floor may be especially weak if you've ever been pregnant, are postmenopausal, do frequent heavy lifting, have been constipated often during your adult life, or are a man with diagnosed prostate problems. The pelvic floor is a large sling of muscles located in your pelvis. This sling starts at your pubic bone in the front and your tailbone in the back, forming an undercarriage or support structure for your entire tummy. Toning your tummy muscles without toning the pelvic floor is like building a house on sand instead of on a firm, solid foundation. The pelvic-floor muscles support and hold in your pelvic organs and abdominal contents. As a side benefit, strong pelvic-floor muscles generally translate to a stronger bladder and more intense sexual awareness.

HOW TO HOLLOW

Use this strategy to hollow your tummy correctly.

1. Lengthen your spine. Try to draw your tailbone away from your neck bone, creating little pockets of space between each vertebra in your spine.
2. Exhale.
3. As you breathe out, draw your tummy inward and upward, bringing your navel in toward your spine and up toward your ribs.

A Test Before You Start

For every movement in the 10-Minute Core Complete routine, I want you to do what physical therapists call hollowing. It involves drawing the navel in toward the spine and up toward your ribs, essentially scooping your abs inward as you firm them. Research completed at James Cook University in Townsville, Australia, shows that this technique will help to support and protect your lower back as well as recruit your transverse abdominis and obliques *during every single exercise in the routine.*

Unfortunately, many people do not use the hollowing technique correctly. Your abdominal muscles may be particularly weak because of a recent pregnancy, the hormonal changes at menopause, excess tummy fat, or lack of use. If this is the case, you may unintentionally pooch your abs or rib cage outward when you try to "suck in your abs."

The difference is subtle but important. If you merely bear downward as you hollow, you'll notice that your tummy appears creased and wrinkled, as if the layers of fat are being pushed outward. This isn't the effect you are looking for! Rather, when you extend and stabilize the spine as you firm your abs, you will see your tummy flatten, appearing smaller—not larger.

To ensure you hollow correctly before and during all of the movements in the routine, I want you to complete the following simple self-assessment. The following four exercises will show you whether you are hollowing or pooching. If, at any of the specified levels, you find yourself pooching, I recommend you put off starting the tummy-specific routine for 1 week, during which time you do these two movements every day. Once you can do level 3 of each movement without pooching, you're ready for the Core Complete routine.

YOU MAY POOCH RATHER THAN HOLLOW IF . . .

- [ ] You have urinary incontinence (leaking urine when you cough, sneeze, or laugh).
- [ ] You have difficulty keeping a tampon in place.
- [ ] You have been diagnosed with a prolapsed vagina.
- [ ] You have ever been pregnant.
- [ ] You are postmenopausal.
- [ ] You have never before trained your abdominal muscles or exercised.

BODY PLANK

A

B

C

Level 1: Get on your forearms and knees in a modi-
fied table position. Firm
your abs, pulling your
tummy up and in toward
your spine without rounding
your back. Imagine that
someone is pulling your
tummy up with a belt. This
small movement will teach
you what "neutral spine"
feels like. You'll want to
keep your spine in a neutral
position for most of the
exercises in the tummy-
specific routine.

Level 2: Using the neutral
spine position that you
learned in Level 1 (with your
tummy pulled up and in
toward your spine but without rounding or overly flat-
tening your back), extend
one leg behind you so that
only the ball of that foot
rests against the floor.
Keep the other knee against
the floor. Hold for 10 seconds and then switch legs.
Continue to alternate legs 5
times on each side.

Level 3: Now you're ready
for a full body plank.
Remember to firm your abs
and use a neutral, long
spine. Place your palms on
the floor under your shoulders and extend both legs
into a pushup position. Try
to lengthen your entire
body, reaching forward
through the crown of your
head and back through your
heels. Hold 10 seconds,
lower your knees to rest,
and repeat for a total of 5
times.

TOWEL PRESS

A

B

C

Level 1: This move will teach you to lengthen your abs as you firm them. Many people who have weak abdominals often firm their abs and pooch them outward, which creates skin and fat rolls—definitely not the effect you are seeking! Instead you want to lengthen through the spine as you firm. To learn how to do so, lie on your back with your knees bent. Place a small, rolled-up towel under your buttocks. Firm your abdominals as you push the small of your back into the floor. The towel will encourage you to lengthen as you firm. Hold for 5 seconds, release, and repeat for a total of 5 times.

Level 2: Do the same exercise but now remove the towel. Place your hand on your tummy to gauge how well you are lengthening as you firm. Your tummy should not pooch outward or crinkle as you firm. Also, your lower ribs should move downward—not up or out. If you see or feel your rib cage rise, return to level 1. Hold 5 seconds, repeating for a total of 5 times.

Level 3: Lie on your back and lift both feet so your thighs form 90-degree angles with your torso and your calves form 90-degree angles with your thighs. Keeping your abdominals firm and long, lower the ball of one foot to the floor at a time, as shown, not allowing your rib cage or lower back to rise. Were you able to do it 5 times on each side without arching your back? Great—then you are ready for the tummy-specific routine!

SIMPLE
HALF SITUP

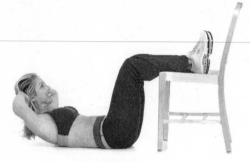

Lie on your back with your knees bent and
heels on a chair. Place your fingertips
behind your head and bend your elbows out
to the sides. Fully relax your back muscles,
and try to keep them relaxed. Without using
your leg or hip muscles, exhale and hollow
your tummy as you crunch up. See if you
can crunch 5 times without feeling any tension in your hips, legs, or back muscles.

CORE CHECK

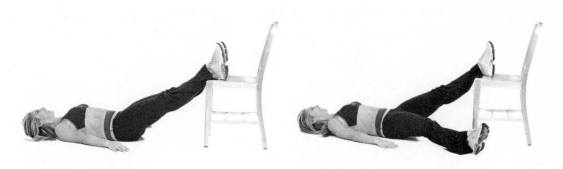

A

Lie on your back with your legs extended and heels on a chair. Rest your arms at your sides, palms facing down. Flatten your back to the floor. Really press it down. Not even a slip of paper should fit between your back and the floor.

B

Then bring your right leg to the right and off the chair, slowly lowering it in a half-circle motion to the floor. Do not allow your lower back to rise as you lower your leg. Lift your right leg, bring it back to the chair, and then repeat with your left leg. Can you do it 3 times on each side without allowing your back to rise?

THE 2-WEEK JUMP-START CORE MOVES PLAN

On this plan, you'll work out 20 to 30 minutes a day, 5 days a week. The Core Moves Plan works in conjunction with the Core Diet Plan. During the 2-week Jump-Start Phase, you will ease yourself into shape. In this way you will gradually progress over time to prevent frustration, soreness, and other common obstacles to exercise.

You will use the following schedule, outlined in more detail in Chapter 12:

* Day 1: 10-Minute Core Complete routine plus 20 minutes of cardio of your choice and 10 1-Minute Fidgetsizers
* Day 2: 20-Minute Core Cardio Blast and 10 1-Minute Fidgetsizers
* Day 3: 20-minute power walk (or cardio of your choice) and 10 1-Minute Fidgetsizers
* Day 4: 10-Minute Core Complete routine plus 20 minutes of cardio of your choice and 10 1-Minute Fidgetsizers
* Day 5: 20-Minute Core Cardio Blast and 10 1-Minute Fidgetsizers
* Day 6: 10 1-Minute Fidgetsizers
* Day 7: 10 1-Minute Fidgetsizers

The 10-Minute Core Complete Routine

The following routine includes the most effective abdominal exercises for strengthening and sculpting your midsection. It's no accident that many of the movements you'll be doing originated from the Pilates method. Research completed at Auburn University in Alabama has determined that Pilates movements more effectively firm the abdomen than standard crunches.

In the following routine, I've also incorporated some moves on the fitness ball, as many studies now show that you use more abdominal muscle fibers to remain stable when you do a crunch on the ball than you would otherwise use when doing a crunch on the floor.

If you're a recovering couch potato who is just starting out, you may notice that your neck hurts when you attempt to do particular crunching-style motions. To reduce this discomfort, try to relax your lower back and neck as much as possible. Tuck your chin in toward your chest to lengthen the back of your neck, and focus on using your abs and not your upper body to lift upward.

SEATED SIDE STRETCH

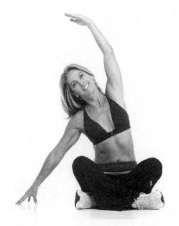

Sit with your legs crossed. Extend your spine from your tailbone through the crown of your head. Inhale as you lift your left arm out to the side and up overhead. Exhale as you reach and bend to the right, feeling the stretch along the left side of your body. Hold for 5 seconds, rise, and repeat on the other side. Continue to switch sides until you've stretched 4 times on each side.

PILATES
BEGINNER
ROLL-UP

Note: If you've recently had a baby, modify this exercise by bending your knees and placing a small, rolled-up towel between your thighs.

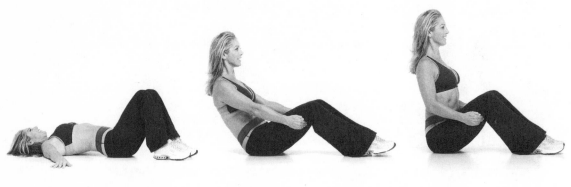

A

For this beginner version of the roll-up, you will bend your knees, lightly using your hands against your thighs to get yourself past any sticking points. Lie on your back with your arms at your sides and your knees bent. Inhale.

B

Exhale as you bring your arms in front of your chest. Engage your abdominals and squeeze your inner thighs together to lift your shoulders, bringing your ribs closer to your hips. As you roll up, let the movement come from your tummy, not from momentum. Grasp your hands against your thighs if needed, as shown. Keep your chin to your chest as you roll up to a sitting position.

C

Sit tall; check that your abs are pulled in toward your spine as you inhale. Exhale and roll back to the starting position, using your abdominals throughout the movement, and try to feel every single vertebra touch the floor one at a time. Complete 3 roll-ups.

The Tummy Type Essentials

LOWER-TUMMY FIRMER

Note: If you've recently had a baby, modify this exercise by doing it with a rolled-up towel hugged between your thighs.

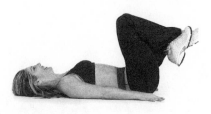

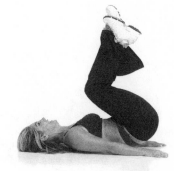

A

Lie on your back. Place your hands near your hips with your palms facing down. Lift your legs, bend your knees, and cross your legs at the ankles.

B

Flatten your shoulders against the floor and draw your abdominals in and up toward your spine. As you exhale, curl your tailbone up, lifting through your lower tummy. Inhale as you lower. Repeat for a total of 4 to 6 times.

STRAIGHT-LEG CRUNCH I

Note: If you've recently had a baby, modify this exercise by doing the crunch with your back against the floor and your knees bent and pressed together.

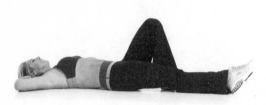

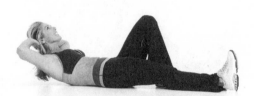

A

B

I love this exercise. By extending one leg, you work your entire midsection, making this one of the most effective abdominal crunches you can do! Lie on your back. Place your hands behind your head with your elbows out to the sides. Bend your left knee and place your left foot against the floor. Extend your right leg.

Flatten your back against the floor and draw your abdominals in and up toward your spine. Exhale as you crunch your head and shoulders up, reaching out through the bottom of the extended leg as you do so. Inhale and lower and repeat 10 to 15 times. Repeat with the left leg extended and right leg bent.

PILATES SINGLE-LEG STRETCH

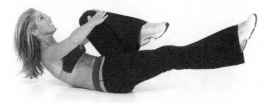

Lie on your back with your knees pulled in toward your chest. Pull your abs toward your spine as you exhale and raise your shoulders from the floor. Bend your left knee to your chest and grab your left calf or ankle with both hands. At the same time, extend your right leg in front of you. Point both feet, drawing both big toes out away from your body. Inhale and switch your legs so that your right leg is near your chest and your left leg is extended. Continue to alternate legs, repeating the entire sequence 5 to 8 times.

LOW HOVER II

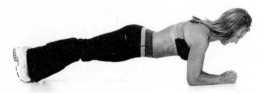

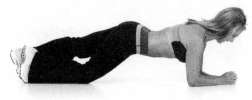

A

This is a fantastic move for your transverse abdominis. Kneel on your hands and knees. Place your forearms on the floor, clasping your hands together. Bring your body weight onto your forearms and balls of your feet. Hold for 30 seconds.

B

Bend your right knee, bringing it toward the floor but not allowing it to touch. Raise it back up and then bend your left. Alternate left and right for 1 minute.

BACK STRENGTHENER I

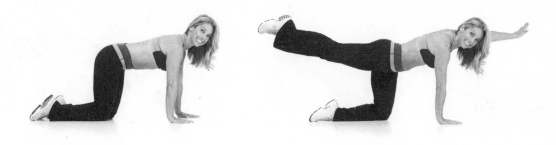

A

In addition to shaping beautiful muscles along your spine, this move also helps you build coordination and balance. Kneel with your knees and palms on the floor, creating a table position with your body.

B

Firm your abdominals as you inhale and simultaneously extend your left arm and right leg, reaching out through your finger-tips and foot. Hold 6 to 8 seconds, breathing normally. Lower, and repeat with the opposite arm and leg. Continue alternating right and left for a total of 5 times on each side.

PILATES
BEGINNER
T-STAND

A

Sit with your right leg extended to the side and your left foot tucked in toward your groin. Place your left hand on the floor beside your buttock.

B

Inhale and use your abdominals to lift your right hip from the floor straight toward the ceiling, sweeping your right arm up toward the ceiling.

C

Exhale as you slowly sweep your right arm forward, extending through your waist and back. Reach your right hand under your body. Feel your upper back open up, fanning open your upper rib cage. Then inhale and use your abs to unfold and lift your torso to the starting position. Repeat 2 more times and then repeat on the opposite side.

The Tummy Type Essentials

SIDE CRUNCH
WITH BALL

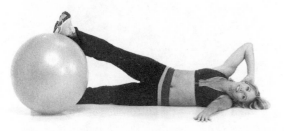 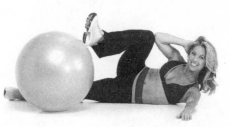

A

Lie on your side with both legs extended to
the side, your right heel on a fitness ball and
your left leg extended just behind the ball.
Rest your extended left arm on the floor at
shoulder level for support. Bend your right
elbow and place your right hand behind your
head for support.

B

Exhale as you lift your head and shoulders,
squeezing through the side of your midsection. As you lift, bend your right knee,
bringing your knee and right elbow toward
each other as you roll the ball in. Lower and
repeat for a total of 10 times. Then switch
sides.

CRUNCH ON BALL

Note: If you've recently had a baby, modify this exercise by doing the crunch with your back against the floor and your knees bent and pressed together.

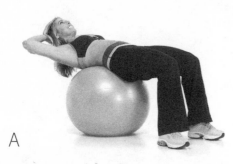

A

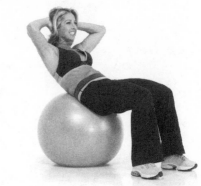

B

Sit on a fitness ball with your knees bent and feet on the floor. Walk your feet forward as you slide your torso down the ball only until your hips start to clear the ball and the very bottom of your lower back presses into the ball. Interlace your fingers behind your head with your elbows out to the sides. Lie back on the ball so that your upper back also rests against it. Then tuck your tailbone in and lift your hips. You should already feel your lower tummy and buttocks firm in this position.

Exhale as you lift your torso, pull your navel in, and firm your abdomen. Imagine that you are curling the bottom of your rib cage and your pelvic bone toward each other, creating a firm arc with your lower body. Keep your chin up as if you were holding an orange between your chin and neck. Inhale as you return to the starting position, lying all the way back on the ball. Do up to 12 repetitions.

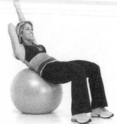

Variation 1

Increase the challenge of this exercise by extending your left arm, grasping your left elbow with your right hand to create a wedge to rest your head against.

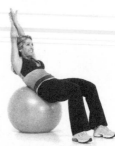

Variation 2

To increase the challenge even more, extend both arms overhead with your palms together.

ROLL-OUT I

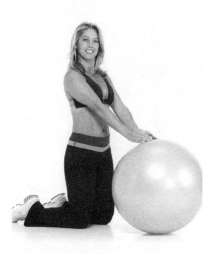

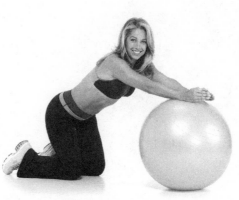

A

Kneel and place the sides of your hands on a fitness ball, with your palms facing each other.

B

Roll the ball away from your torso as you extend your arms, keeping your hips over your knees. Return to the starting position and repeat for a total of 5 to 10 times.

TORSO TRIMMER

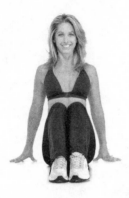

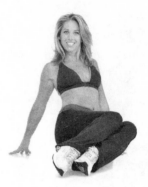

A

Sit with your knees bent and feet on the floor. Place your palms on the floor by your sides.

B

Lower your knees to the floor to the left. Bring them back to center and then lower them to the right. Continue alternating right and left for 1 minute.

SEATED CHEST STRETCH

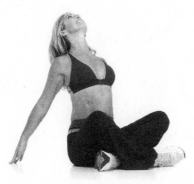

Sit with your legs crossed. Lift up through your breastbone as you reach your arms behind you, pressing your fingertips into the floor behind your buttocks to feel a stretch in your chest. Hold for 15 seconds. Release.

The 20-Minute Core Cardio Blast

I'm confident that you'll love this 20-minute heart-pumping, core-sculpting total-body workout. It's one of the most efficient and effective workout routines I've ever designed. Because you'll use light hand weights during this routine, I recommend you wear shoes. Wear any type of comfortable clothing (something that moves with you). You can do the routine anywhere—really. Outside while watching your kids in the yard (just bring yourself, your hand weights, and a mat for your comfort) . . . inside in front of the TV . . . at a friend's house . . . at the gym . . . in a hotel room. Don't let your location stop you from moving. The routine requires just a small amount of floor space (you'll need roughly a 6- by 6-foot square of space).

This routine includes three exercise elements that work like an effective 1-2-3 punching combination to knock out tummy fat for good.

1. **Cardio:** I've interspersed 3 minutes of cardio-revving movements throughout the routine to get and keep your heart rate up as you tone your muscles from head to toe. Cardio is one of the fastest and most effective ways to burn tummy fat.
2. **Weight training:** You'll use light hand weights to build muscle all over your body to kick up your metabolism 24/7.
3. **Core building:** When you combine cardio with weights into one heart-pumping, muscle-sculpting workout, you get serious results in record time. The following routine does even more. It also builds core strength—in your abs, sides, and back—with just about every single move. Many moves include challenging combinations that will test your body's balance and agility. Keeping your body surprised like this will simultaneously firm your core muscles as the routine strengthens your arms, shoulders, chest, back, and legs.

WARMUP
STANDING
STRETCH

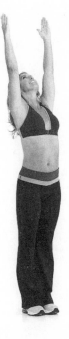

Stand with your feet under your hips. Inhale
deeply as you reach your arms overhead.
Reach down through the bottoms of your
feet and up through the crown of your head
and fingertips as you lengthen your entire
body. Release and repeat 1 time.

WARMUP
STANDING SIDE
STRETCH

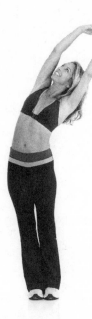

From the warmup standing stretch, clasp
your hands together overhead and bend to
the left, feeling a stretch along the right side
of your torso. Inhale as you return to center
and then repeat to the right.

FRONT JAB

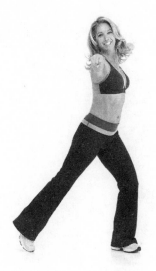

Stand with your feet under your hips. Step to
the left with your left foot as you throw a
jab, as shown, toward an imaginary opponent in front of you with your right arm. Step
your feet back together as you bring your
arm back. Then repeat to the left. Continue
alternating sides for 1 minute.

MAMBO

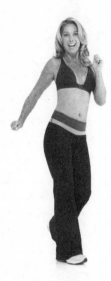

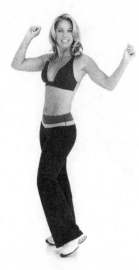

A

B

Step forward with your right leg as you swing your hip out to the right.

Then step back with your right leg, swinging your hip to the right as you place your foot. Do this for 30 seconds with your right foot and then repeat with your left leg.

BASKETBALL SHUFFLE

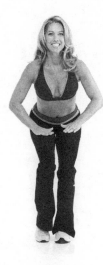

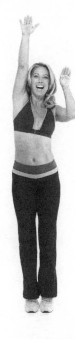

A

Stand with your legs under your hips, your knees slightly bent. Shuffle to the right 3 to 4 steps (depending on your exercise space) as you dribble an imaginary basketball.

B

Bring both feet under your hips, bend your knees, squat down, and then spring upward as you shoot your imaginary ball to the hoop. Land and shuffle back to the left, alternating left and right for 1 minute.

SQUAT
WITH SHOULDER
SHAPER

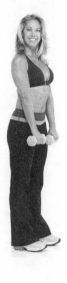

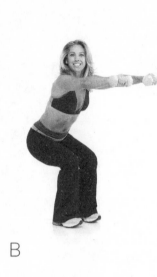

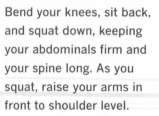

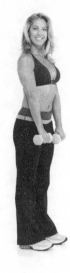

A

B

C

Stand with your feet slightly wider than shoulder width apart. Grasp a pair of light hand weights. Rest your hands in front of your thighs, your arms extended.

Bend your knees, sit back, and squat down, keeping your abdominals firm and your spine long. As you squat, raise your arms in front to shoulder level.

Press into your heels as you straighten your legs and lower your arms. Repeat for a total of 15 times.

LUNGE
WITH CHEST FLY I

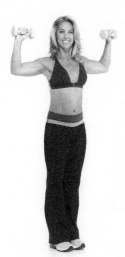

A

Stand with your feet under your hips. Grasp a pair of light hand weights and extend your elbows out to the sides at shoulder level, your arms bent at right angles.

B

Step back with your right foot and bend both knees, sinking down into a lunge with both legs bent at 90-degree angles. As you sink into the lunge, bring your elbows together in front of your chest in a pressing motion. Step back to the starting position as you open your elbows out to the sides. Repeat by stepping back with your left foot. Continue alternating legs for 10 lunges on each side.

LUNGE
WITH SIDE CHOP

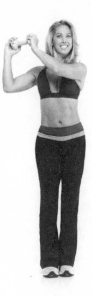

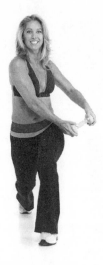

A

Grasp one dumbbell with both hands. Stand with your feet under your hips. Extend your arms above your right shoulder, holding the dumbbell sideways, as shown.

B

Step back with your right foot, bend both knees at right angles, and bring your arms forward and down over your left knee, as if you were chopping wood. Step back to the starting position as you raise your arms. Repeat for a total of 5 times and then switch sides.

The Tummy Type Essentials

TRICEPS TONER

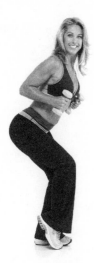

A

Stand with your feet under your hips. Grasp a pair of light hand weights with your elbows bent. Bend your knees and lift your right heel.

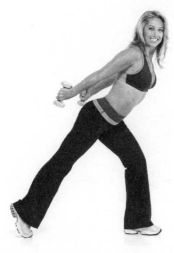

B

Step back with your right leg, bringing your legs into a scissors position. Bend your left knee, but keep your right leg extended, allowing your right heel to lift. Lean forward slightly and extend your arms toward the floor. Keeping your arms close to your body, lift them behind you to tone the tops of your arms. Step back to the starting position, alternating between positions A and B 10 times before switching legs.

JUMP ROPE

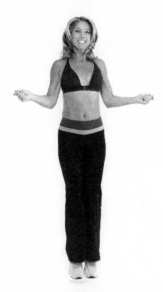

You don't need a real jump rope to reap the calorie-burning benefits of this exercise! Just jump up and down as you pretend to swing a rope. Do this for 1 minute.

SQUAT KNEE LIFT

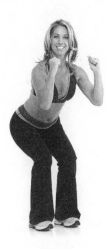

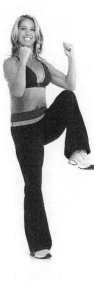

A

Stand with your feet under your hips. Bend your knees and squat down, sitting back into your buttocks.

B

Then extend your legs. Just as they straighten, lift your left knee to your chest. Then lower your left leg, squat down, and raise your right knee. Continue alternating squats and knee lifts up for 1 minute.

CHA-CHA

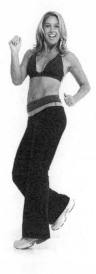

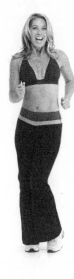

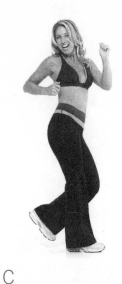

A

This famous Latin dance will keep you moving! Start with your feet under your hips. Step forward and slightly to the right with your left foot, swiveling your hips as you do so.

B

Step your feet back under your hips, swiveling them again to a "cha cha cha" cadence.

C

Then do the same to the left, as if your feet were chasing each other. Do the cha-cha for 1 minute.

PLIÉ SQUAT
WITH BICEPS
CURL I

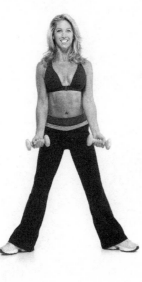

A

Stand with your feet slightly wider than
shoulder width apart. Turn your toes out and
heels in. Grasp a pair of dumbbells, keeping
your arms straight, with your hands resting
in front of your thighs and palms facing out.

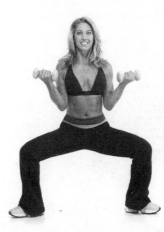

B

Bend your knees out to the sides as you
drop your tailbone and squat down. At the
same time, curl your hands toward your
upper arms. Rise and repeat for a total of
10 times.

The Core Moves

DEADLIFT
INTO DOUBLE-ARM
ROW

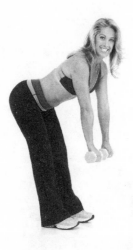

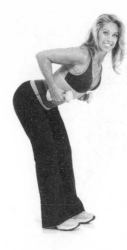

A

Stand with your feet under your hips. Grasp a pair of light hand weights, resting your arms at your sides. Bend forward from the hips and extend your arms toward the floor so they end up directly below your shoulders, as shown.

B

Lift your elbows toward the ceiling, keeping your arms close to your ribs. Lower your hands toward the floor, rise to the starting position, and repeat for a total of 10 times.

STANDING
PILATES
SWIMMING

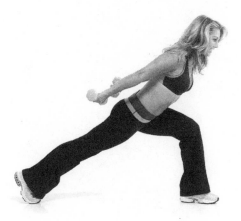

Stand with your feet under your hips. Grasp
a pair of light hand weights. Take a large
step back with your right leg, bending your
left knee, leaning forward, and placing your
palms against the floor in a runner's lunge.
Lift your arms and upper body off the floor
and bring your extended arms to your sides
with your palms facing up. Pulse your palms
up toward the ceiling, mimicking a swimming motion. Do this up to 15 seconds, and
then switch legs and repeat.

MARCHING
IN PLACE

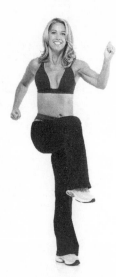

With your feet under your hips, march,
bringing your knees as high as possible.
If you want to burn more calories, consider
jogging in place instead. Do this for
1 minute.

JUMPING JACKS

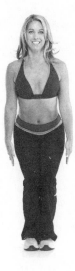

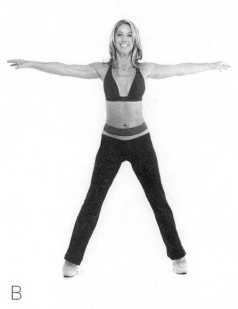

A

Start with your feet under your hips and hands down at your sides.

B

Jump your feet out to the sides into a wide angle as you simultaneously lift your arms laterally out to the sides. Jump back in as you lower your arms. Repeat for 1 minute.

KNEE BEND WITH OVERHEAD REACH

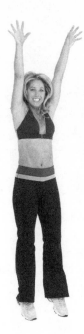

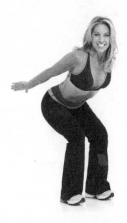

A

Stand with your feet under your hips. All in one motion, bend your knees and sit back into a squat as you lower your arms.

B

Then straighten your legs as you raise your arms overhead and jump, as shown, into the air before landing and completing another squat. Repeat for 1 minute.

PUSHUP I

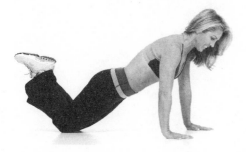

A

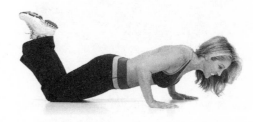

B

In phase 1, you'll build strength in your upper body and core by doing pushups on your knees. In phase 2, you'll advance to doing them on your toes. For the phase 1 version, kneel and place your palms on the floor so that your body forms a straight line from your knees to your head. Lift your feet and shins.

Bend your elbows out to the sides as you lower your chest to the floor, keeping our abdominals firm and your back flat. Do 3 to 5 repetitions.

PILATES
CRISSCROSS I

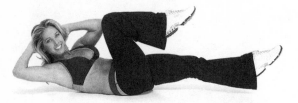

Lie on your back with your head resting into your fingertips. Open your elbows to the sides. Bend your knees, placing your feet flat on the floor. Firm your abdominals and lift both feet off the floor. Exhale as you extend your left leg and simultaneously bring your right knee toward your chest. At the same time, rotate your shoulders, bringing your left elbow toward your right knee. Once your shoulder almost reaches the floor, exhale and repeat the move by extending your right leg and bringing your left knee in toward your chest. Repeat the sequence 5 to 8 times.

The Tummy Type Essentials

REVERSE CRUNCH

Note: If you've recently had a baby, do this exercise with a small towel between your thighs.

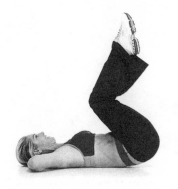

A

Lie on your back. Place your hands behind your head. Bend your knees and lift your feet off the floor.

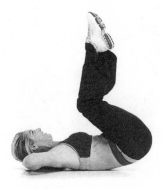

B

Flatten your back against the floor and draw your abdominals in and up toward your spine. As you exhale, curl your tailbone up, lifting through your lower tummy. Repeat for a total of 5 to 8 times.

PLANK I

Note: If you've recently had a baby, do this exercise by hugging a rolled-up towel or small ball or pillow between your thighs.

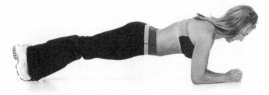

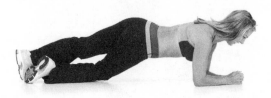

A

Kneel, place your elbows and forearms on the floor, and clasp your hands. Straighten your legs so you are supporting your body weight on the balls of your feet and your forearms.

B

Lower your right knee to the floor, bringing it down and slightly to the left. Just as it grazes the floor, lift it back to the starting position. Alternate dropping the right and left knee for 10 total repetitions.

SWAN

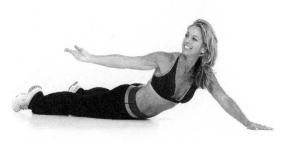

Lie on your tummy with your arms extended
in front of your head. Without pressing into
the floor with your hands, use your upper
back muscles to lift your chest and upper
tummy off the floor. Lift your right hand and
rotate your torso to the right, as shown.
Return to center, lower your chest to the
floor, and then repeat on the other side.
Complete 3 repetitions on each side.

BUTT KICK

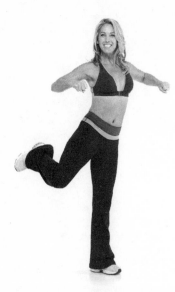

Standing with your feet slightly wider than shoulder width apart, shift your weight onto your left leg as you lift your right foot toward your right buttock. As you do so, pull your elbows back behind your torso. Lower your leg and your arms and repeat with the other leg. Continue alternating legs for 1 minute.

FRONT TAP

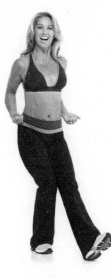

Stand with your feet under your hips and
your knees slightly bent. Step forward with
your left foot, tapping your left heel to the
floor. Step back and then step forward with
your right heel, continuing to alternate sides
for 1 minute.

LEG LIFT

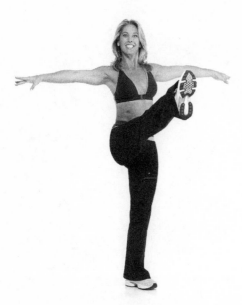

Starting with your feet under your hips and
arms extended to your sides from your
shoulders, lift your right leg in front as high
as you can. Lower and repeat with your left
leg. Continue to alternate legs for 1 minute.

FORWARD BEND

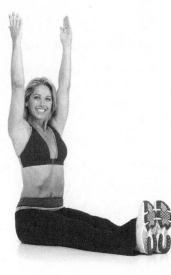

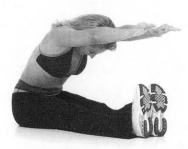

A

Sit with your legs extended. Raise your arms overhead.

B

Reach your arms out from your shoulders. Exhale as you bend forward and reach for your toes. Hold for 15 seconds. Release.

THE KEEP-ON-LOSING CORE MOVES ROUTINES

You're fitter now than you were 2 weeks ago, so it's time to turn up the heat on your workouts. In this section, you'll find a new 10-Minute Core Complete routine and 20-Minute Core Cardio Blast. These routines mirror the routines you've completed during the past 2 weeks. To make this transition to the Keep-On-Losing Phase as seamless as possible, I've included many of the same moves you've grown accustomed to, only in this phase, you'll challenge yourself with some intermediate and advanced variations. You'll also find a few additional exercises not included in the Jump-Start Phase. The addition of these new movements will help to challenge your body in new ways—ensuring your long-term success.

You'll follow the same exercise schedule you did during phase 1, working out 5 days a week, but you will add more cardio to the mix. Your weekly schedule looks like this.

* Day 1: 10-Minute Core Complete routine plus 25 minutes of cardio of your choice and 10 1-Minute Fidgetsizers
* Day 2: 25-Minute Core Cardio Blast and 10 1-Minute Fidgetsizers
* Day 3: 25-minute power walk (or cardio of your choice) and 10 1-Minute Fidgetsizers
* Day 4: 10-Minute Core Complete routine plus 25 minutes of cardio of your choice and 10 1-Minute Fidgetsizers
* Day 5: 25-Minute Core Cardio Blast and 10 1-Minute Fidgetsizers
* Day 6: 10 1-Minute Fidgetsizers
* Day 7: 10 1-Minute Fidgetsizers

To increase your success even more, I recommend you do something fun and active on your days off from official movement. Play actively with your children, take a hike at a nearby park, or go for a bike ride. Enjoy the outdoors and continue to work toward becoming a mover rather than a sitter!

10-Minute Core Complete Routine (Keep-On-Losing Phase)

The following routine should look and feel familiar to you. You did versions of many of these exercises in phase 1. Now you'll turn up the heat on those abs with a few additional moves as well as more challenging variations of the movements you completed during phase 1. If any move feels too challenging for you, use the phase 1 variation of that move (or omit the move altogether) until you build your fitness.

SEATED SIDE STRETCH

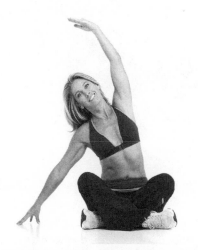

Sit with your legs crossed. Extend your spine from your tailbone through the crown of your head. Inhale as you lift your left arm out to the side and up overhead. Exhale as your reach and bend to the right, feeling the stretch along the left side of your body. Hold for 5 seconds, rise, and repeat on the other side. Continue to switch sides until you've stretched 4 times on each side.

HEEL TAP

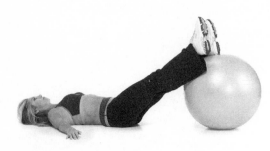

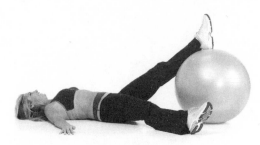

A

This simple exercise will help you develop stability through your midsection as you strengthen your transverse abdominis muscle. Lie on your back. Place your hands on the floor by your sides, palms down. Lift your legs and place your heels on top of a fitness ball.

B

Lift your right heel an inch off the ball and trace the curve of the ball with your heel, lowering your right foot and leg to the floor to your right. Lightly tap the floor and then lift your leg back to the starting position. As you move, try to keep your hips and back stationary. Don't allow the slightest wiggle! Repeat with the left leg. Continue alternating right and left for a total of 10 repetitions.

LOWER-TUMMY
AND PELVIC-FLOOR
STRENGTHENER
ON THE BALL

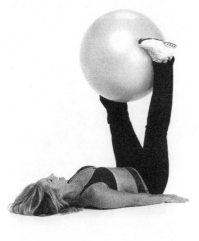

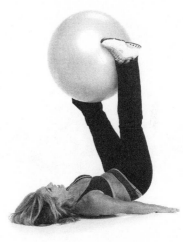

A

Rest your hands at your sides and hug a fitness ball between your thighs, knees, and
feet. Simply hugging the ball to keep it in
place will activate your inner thighs and your
pelvic-floor muscles—and you haven't even
done a crunch yet!

B

Flatten your shoulders against the floor and
draw your abdominals in and up toward your
spine. As you exhale, curl your tailbone up,
lifting through your lower tummy, not allowing the ball to fall out from your legs. Lower
and repeat for a total of 10 times.

STRAIGHT-LEG
CRUNCH II

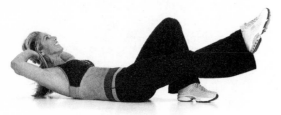
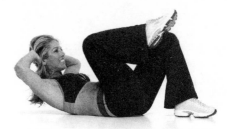

A

You completed a version of this exercise during phase 1. Now that you've built some strength, you're ready to increase the challenge by lifting your extended leg. Lie on your back. Place your hands behind your head with your elbows out to the sides. Bend your left knee and place your left foot against the floor. Extend your right leg and lift it a few inches off the floor. Flatten your back against the floor and draw your abdominals in and up toward your spine. Exhale as you crunch your head and shoulders up, just until you bring your shoulder blades off the floor, as shown.

B

Crunch your upper body up a little bit higher (as high as you can) as you bring your right knee in toward your face. Return to the starting position and repeat for a total of 10 to 15 times. Repeat with the left leg extended and right leg bent.

PILATES FULL T-STAND

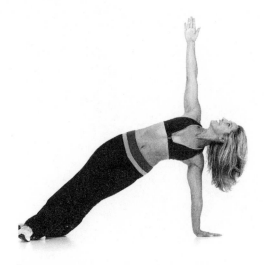

A

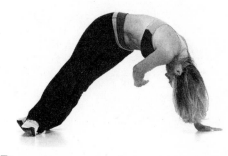

B

You practiced one version of the T-stand during phase 1 of the program. Let's increase the challenge by extending your bottom leg. Sit with your right leg extended to the side and your left foot tucked in toward your groin. Extend both legs to the right and then use your abs as you inhale and press through your left hand and lift through your right hip. You should form the letter T with your body.

Exhale as you slowly sweep your right arm forward, extending through your waist and back. Reach your right hand under your body and toward your left. Feel your upper back open up, fanning open your upper rib cage. Then exhale and use your abs to unfold and raise your torso to the starting position. Repeat 2 more times on your right side and then repeat on the opposite side.

BACK
STRENGTHENER II

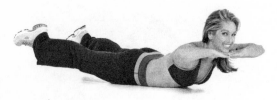

Lie on your tummy with your legs extended.
Bend your elbows and place your fingertips
under your chin. Lengthen your entire body
from your head to your toes. Then lift your
legs and upper torso, as shown. Hold 5 seconds, lower, and repeat up to 3 times.

WAISTLINE
SLIMMER

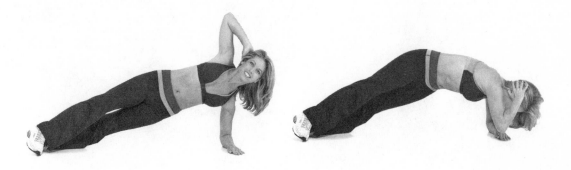

A

Lie on your left side. Bend your left elbow
and place your left forearm against the floor.
Stack your feet on top of each other. Lift
your torso, balancing your body weight on
your left forearm and side of your left foot,
as shown. Bend your right elbow and place
your right palm behind your head.

B

Keeping your hips lifted as high as possible,
bring your right elbow down toward your left
hand. Then return to the starting position
and repeat 3 to 5 times before switching
sides.

PILATES DOUBLE-LEG STRETCH

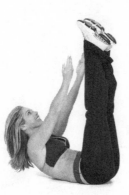

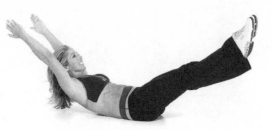

A

During phase 1, you built abdominal strength with the Pilates single-leg stretch. Now you're ready to up the ante by extending both legs simultaneously. I love this exercise because it works the entire front of the tummy! Lie on your back with your legs extended toward the ceiling. Inhale as you use your abdominals to lift your shoulders off the floor, reaching your hands toward your feet.

B

Exhale as you press your arms and legs out, as shown, making sure to engage and move from your abs. Extend through your fingertips and toes. Inhale as you bring your knees back toward your chest and your arms back toward your knees. Repeat for a total of 5 to 8 times.

WAISTLINE CHOP ON THE BALL

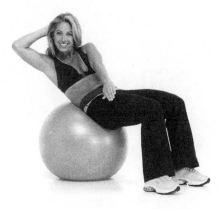

This new phase 2 exercise will help to whittle that waistline! Sit on a fitness ball with your knees bent and feet on the floor. Walk your feet forward as you slide your torso down the ball just until your hips start to clear the ball and the very bottom of your lower back presses into the ball. Interlace your fingers behind your head with your elbows out to the sides. Lie back on the ball so that your upper back also rests against the ball. Then tuck your tailbone in and lift your hips. You should already feel your lower tummy and buttocks firm in this position. Exhale as you lift your torso, as if you were going to do a crunch. Rather than crunching straight up, however, extend your left arm toward your right knee, as shown, as if you were swinging an axe. Inhale as you return to the starting position, repeating with the opposite arm. Do 12 total repetitions.

TUMMY TUCK

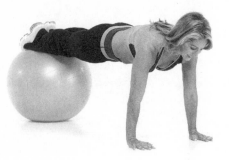

A

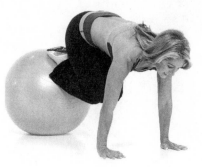

B

This challenging, new phase 2 exercise will strengthen your entire core. Start in a pushup position with your shins on a fitness ball and your hands on the floor under your chest. (*Note:* Positioning the ball so that your thighs are against it will make the exercise a little easier; placing the tops of your feet on the ball will make it harder.) Firm your abdominals and lift your hips so that your back is flat.

Exhale as you tuck your knees in toward your chest, moving the ball along the floor as you do so. Inhale as you return to the starting position. Continue to tuck and then uncoil up to 12 times.

ROLL-OUT II

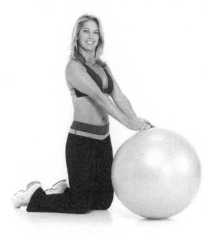

A

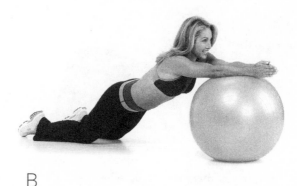

B

You did one version of the roll-out in phase 1. Now you will increase the challenge of this move by rolling the ball farther away and bringing your hips forward of your knees. To start, kneel and place the sides of your hands on the ball, with your palms facing each other.

Roll the ball out from you as you extend your arms, this time allowing your hips to come forward until you feel your abdominals tighten. Come as far forward as you feel comfortable, even bringing your forearms onto the fitness ball if possible, as shown. Repeat 5 to 10 times. This full extension will work your lats in your back as well as your abdominals.

YOGA BRIDGE STRETCH

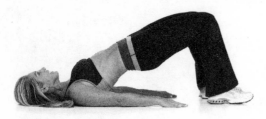

Lie on your back with your knees bent and your feet flat on the floor. Rest your arms at your sides with your palms down and at about hip level. Take a deep breath. Exhale as you firm your abs and curl your hips up to feel a stretch in your chest and tummy, as shown. Hold for 15 seconds and then roll down one vertebra at a time.

REVERSE PLANK STRETCH

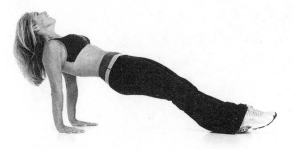

Sit with your legs extended in front and your palms at your sides near your buttocks. Exhale, press into your palms, and then straighten your arms as you lift your body. Your forehead, shoulders, hips, and heels should form a straight line, as shown. Keep your shoulder blades pushed back and low on your back, your chest open, your neck long, and imagine that a string is lifting your chest to the ceiling. Hold for 10 to 15 seconds and then rest.

The 25-Minute Core Cardio Blast (Keep-On-Losing Phase)

Are you ready to burn fat, build muscle, and firm your tummy even more? This Core Cardio Blast builds on the routine you completed in phase 1. I know how frustrating it is to try to learn a new exercise routine so soon after *finally* getting the hang of the one you've been doing. That's why many of the cardio moves in this routine are either the same as what you did during phase 1 or slightly more challenging. To keep things interesting, I've also incorporated some new moves that I'm confident you will find challenging, invigorating, and fun. Expect this routine to take you a little more time—about 5 to 10 minutes more— than your phase 1 routine. I'm confident you'll decide that the extra time is well worth it!

WARMUP STANDING STRETCH

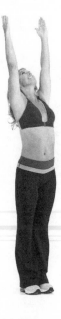

Stand with your feet under your hips. Inhale deeply as you reach your arms overhead. Reach down through the bottoms of your feet and up through the crown of your head and fingertips as you lengthen your entire body. Release.

WARMUP
STANDING
SIDE STRETCH

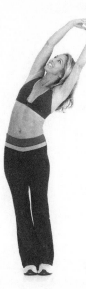

From the warmup standing stretch, clasp
your hands together overhead and bend to
the left, feeling a stretch along the right side
of your torso. Inhale as you return to center
and then repeat to the right. Release.

UPPERCUTS

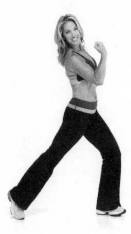

Stand with your feet under your hips. Step to
the left with your left foot as you throw an
uppercut, as shown. To throw an uppercut,
keep your elbow in close to your body and
drive your fist upward, as if you were trying
to punch someone underneath the chin.
Throw uppercuts to both sides, alternating
for 1 minute.

SQUAT WITH KICK

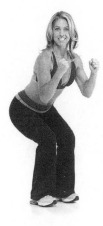

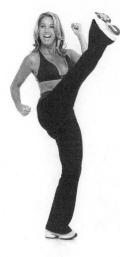

A

Stand with your feet under your hips and your elbows bent in a boxing stance. Bend your knees and sit back into a squat, keeping your back long and flat.

B

Extend your legs back to standing, lift your right knee to your chest, and then kick forward, as if you were trying to kick an opponent in the chin, as shown. Lower your leg to standing, do another squat, and this time kick with your left leg. Continue alternating right and left for 1 minute.

ABDOMINAL PULL

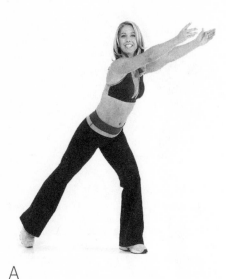

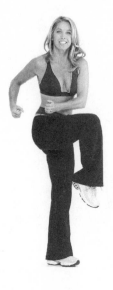

A

B

Stand with your feet under your hips. Step to the left and slightly forward with your left foot and extend your arms overhead and to the left, as if you were trying to reach an object on a high shelf.

Pull your hands down toward the right side of your waist as you simultaneously lift your right knee to your chest. Repeat for 30 seconds on this side before switching legs.

SIDE LUNGE WITH OVERHEAD PRESS

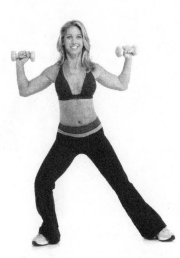

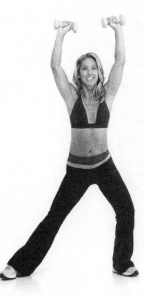

A

Stand with your feet slightly wider than hip width apart. Grasp dumbbells in each hand. Raise your arms, bringing your elbows to shoulder height. Bend your elbows at 90-degree angles. Bend your right knee and squat down, as shown, keeping your left leg extended.

B

Switch sides, bending your left knee and extending your right. As you do so, raise your arms overhead. Alternate sides, completing a total of 7 repetitions on each side.

LUNGE
WITH CHEST FLY II

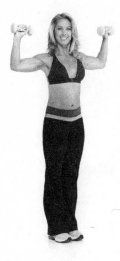

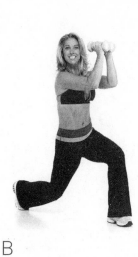

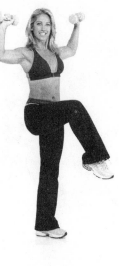

A

You did a version of this exercise in phase 1. Now you'll do the move with one leg off the ground to challenge your ability to stay balanced. Stand with your feet under your hips. Grasp a pair of light hand weights and extend your elbows out to the sides at shoulder level, your arms bent at right angles.

B

Step back with your right foot and bend both knees, sinking down into a lunge with both legs bent at 90-degree angles. As you lower into the lunge, bring your elbows together in front of your chest in a pressing motion.

C

Open your elbows back out to the sides as you begin to lift your right knee up toward your chest. Do a total of 10 lunges, and then switch legs; make sure to control your core.

SIDE LUNGE WITH LATERAL RAISE

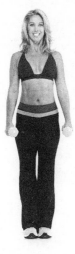

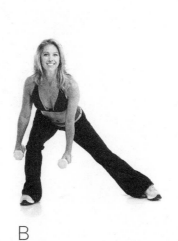

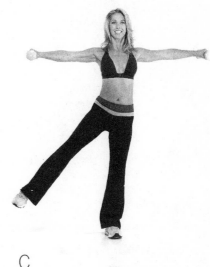

A

You completed a similar exercise during phase 1 but will increase the challenge in phase 2 by adding a side leg lift. Grasp a dumbbell in each hand. Stand with your feet under your hips and your arms at your sides.

B

Step to the right with your right leg, bending your right knee and bending forward from the hips, dangling your hands toward the floor, as shown.

C

Return to an upright position. As you fully extend your legs, shift your body weight into your left leg, raising your right leg out to the side as you simultaneously lift your arms laterally out to the sides to shoulder level. Return to standing and repeat, alternating the side squat with the side leg lift a total of 6 times before switching sides.

TRICEPS TONER

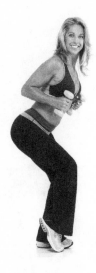

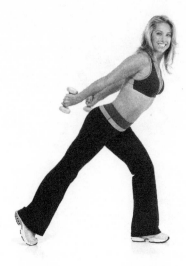

A

You completed this move during phase 1. The phase 2 version is no different. Stand with your feet under your hips. Grasp a pair of light hand weights with your elbows bent. Bend your knees and lift your right heel.

B

Step back with your right leg, bringing your legs into a scissors position. Bend your left knee, but keep your right leg extended, allowing your right heel to lift. Lean forward slightly and extend your arms toward the floor. Keeping your arms close to your body, lift them behind you to tone the tops of your arms. Step back to the starting position, alternating between positions A and B for a total of 10 times before switching legs.

JUMP ROPE

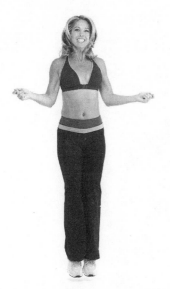

You need not use a real jump rope to reap the calorie-burning benefits of this exercise! Just jump up and down as you pretend to swing a rope. Jump for $1\frac{1}{2}$ minutes.

KNEE-UP

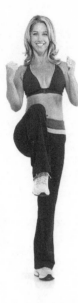

A

Stand with your feet under your hips. Lift your right knee to your chest, as shown. Lower your right foot to the floor and then lift your left knee to your chest.

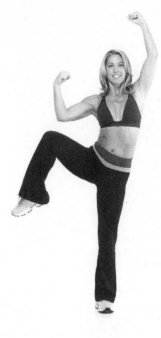

B

As you plant your left foot, lift your right knee again, this time lifting it to the side, as shown. Lower and repeat with your left leg. Continue alternating front and sides with both legs for 1 minute.

LATERAL
BOUNDING

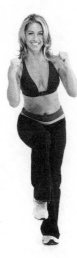

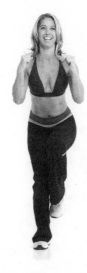

A

B

Stand with your feet under your hips. Take a big jump to the left, as if you were jumping to the left square of a four-square.

Then jump back to the right. Continue bounding from one side to the other for 1 minute. *Note:* If you get too winded to keep it up for a full minute or your joints can't take the high impact, simply step from one side to the other, taking very large steps and bringing your knee up to your chest before you step out.

PLIÉ SQUAT
WITH BICEPS
CURL II

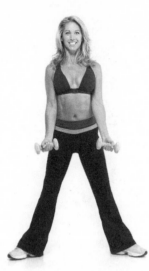

A

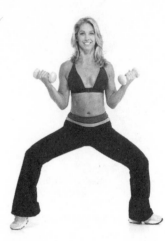

B

Stand with your feet slightly wider than shoulder width apart. Turn your toes out and heels in. Grasp a pair of dumbbells, keeping your arms straight, with your hands resting in front of your thighs and palms facing out.

Bend your knees out to the sides as you drop your tailbone and squat down, lifting your right heel and coming onto the ball of your right foot. You should feel an extra firming in your inner thighs. At the same time, curl your hands toward your upper arms. Lower your heel, rise, and repeat, this time raising your left heel. Complete 10 repetitions on each side.

DEADLIFT
INTO DOUBLE-ARM ROW

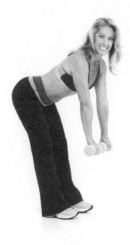

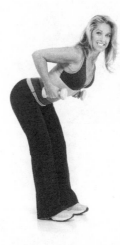

A

B

Stand with your feet under your hips. Grasp a pair of light hand weights, resting your arms at your sides. Bend forward from the hips and extend your arms toward the floor so they end up directly below your shoulders, as shown.

Lift your elbows toward the ceiling, keeping your arms close to your ribs. Lower your hands toward the floor, rise to the starting position, and repeat for a total of 10 times. Keep your abs strong, back flat, and knees slightly bent.

STANDING
PILATES
SWIMMING

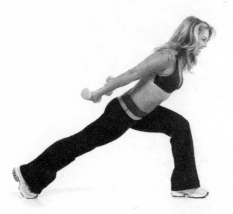

Stand with your feet under your hips. Grasp
light weights in your hands. Take a large
step back with your right leg, bending your
left knee, leaning forward, and placing your
palms against the floor in a runner's lunge.
Lift your arms and upper body off the floor
and bring your extended arms to your sides
with your palms facing up. Pulse your palms
up toward the ceiling, mimicking a swimming motion. Do this up to 15 seconds, and
then switch legs and repeat.

PUSHUP II

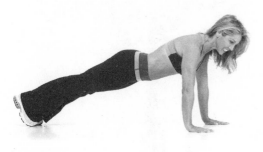

A

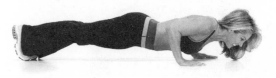

B

In phase 1, you did pushups with your knees on the ground. Now challenge yourself, trying them with your legs extended. Do as many as you can this way and then lower your knees, returning to the phase 1 version for as many reps as possible. To do the phase 2 version, place your palms on the floor and extend your legs, so that your body forms a straight line from your toes to your head.

Bend your elbows out to the sides as you lower your chest to the floor, keeping your abdomen firm and your back flat. Do 3 to 5 total reps.

SIDE KICK

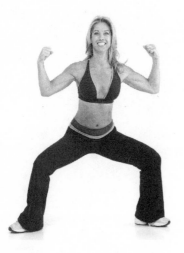

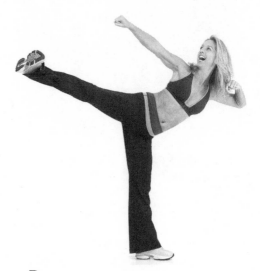

A

Stand with your feet slightly wider than shoulder width apart. Turn your toes out and heels in. Bend your knees and sit back into a squat, as shown. Raise your arms out to your sides and bend your elbows (in a "look how strong I am" posture).

B

Straighten your knees, center your body weight over your left leg, and then kick your right leg out to the side as you punch to the side with your right arm. Return to standing and alternate squatting with kicking on each side for $1\frac{1}{2}$ minutes.

SIDE TWIST

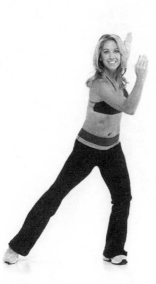

A

With your legs still in a wide stance and your arms raised with elbows bent from the previous exercise, bend your left knee as you twist your torso to the left, as shown.

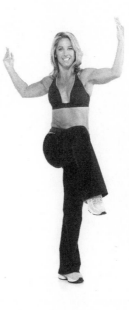

B

Untwist your torso back to face front as you simultaneously lift your right knee to your chest. Continue twisting to the left and raising your right knee for 45 seconds, and then switch sides.

JUMPING JACKS

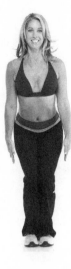

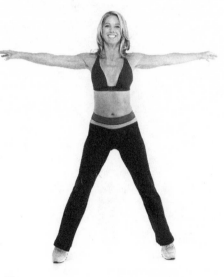

A

Start with your feet under your hips and hands down at your sides.

B

Jump your feet out to the sides into a wide angle as you simultaneously lift your arms laterally out to the sides. Jump back in as you lower your arms. Repeat for 1$\frac{1}{2}$ minutes.

PILATES CRISSCROSS II

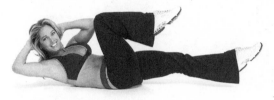

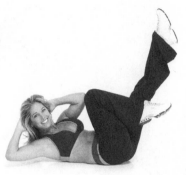

A

Lie on your back with your head resting into your fingertips. Open your elbows to the sides. Bend your knees, placing your feet flat on the floor. Firm your abdominals and lift both feet off the floor. Exhale as you extend your left leg and simultaneously bring your right knee toward your chest. At the same time, rotate your shoulders, bringing your left elbow toward your right knee.

B

Then lift your left leg up about 2 to 3 feet. Lower and change positions, repeating the move by extending your right leg and bringing your left knee in toward your chest. Repeat the entire sequence 5 to 8 times total.

ROLL-OVER

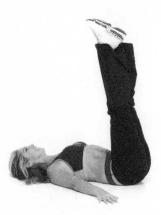

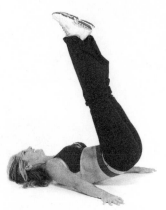

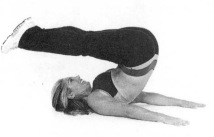

A

Lie on your back. Rest your arms by your sides with your palms facing down. Extend your legs toward the ceiling.

B

Lift your tailbone and slowly roll up, lifting your buttocks and lower back off the mat. Keep your feet pointed.

C

Once you've lifted as far as you can go, flex your feet, reaching out through the bottoms of your feet as you slowly roll back down. Repeat for a total of 5 times.

PLANK II

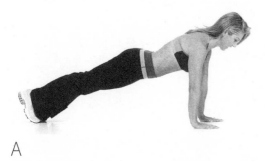

A

Get into a pushup position, with your hands under your chest and your legs extended, supporting your body weight on the balls of your feet and your hands.

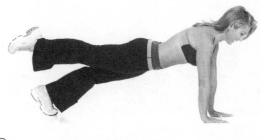

B

Lift your right leg, as shown. With your right leg up, shift your body weight forward a few inches. Then, shift your weight back, lower your leg, and repeat on the other side. Complete 3 reps on each side.

SUPERMAN

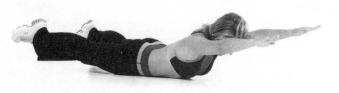

Lie on your tummy with your arms and legs
extended. Inhale as you lift your arms, upper
body, and legs, creating length through your
spine. Hold 10 seconds, release, and repeat
1 time.

BUTT KICK

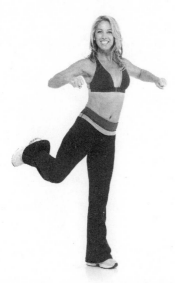

Standing with your feet slightly wider than
shoulder width apart, shift your weight onto
your left leg as you lift your right foot toward
your right buttock. As you do so, pull your
elbows back behind your torso. Lower your
leg and your arms and repeat with the
other leg. Continue alternating legs for
1½ minutes.

FRONT TAP

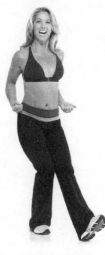

Stand with your feet under your hips and
your knees slightly bent. Step forward with
your left foot, tapping your left heel to the
floor. Step back and then step forward with
your right heel, continuing to alternate sides
for 1½ minutes.

SIDE LEG KICK

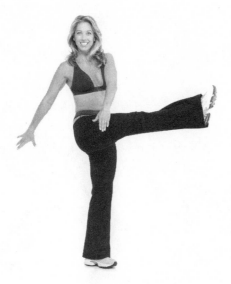

Stand with your feet under your hips and
your arms extended in front at chest level.
Shift your body weight to your left leg as you
lift your right leg forward and to the left. At
the same time, lower your arms down and to
the right, twisting through your torso as you
do so. Lower your leg, raise your arms, and
repeat on the other side. Continue alternating sides for 1 minute. Feel like you're on
Broadway.

PLANK
INTO DOWN DOG

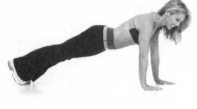 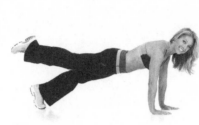 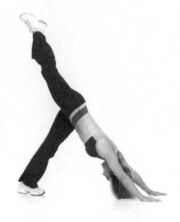

A

Kneel, placing your palms on the floor, and then extend your legs so that your body forms a straight line from your feet to your head. Reach out through the top of your head and your heels to create length in your body. Keep your shoulders relaxed, your shoulder blades low on your back.

B

Lift your right foot as high as you can. Hold for 15 to 30 seconds.

C

Press into your hands as you lift your hips toward the ceiling, forming a triangle with your body. Keep your right leg extended and lifted as high as you can, but don't allow your right hip to rise higher than your left. Hold for 15 to 30 seconds. Lower and then repeat with the left leg lifted. Complete 2 repetitions on each side.

FORWARD BEND

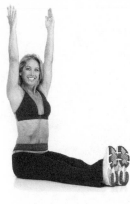

A

Sit with your legs extended. Raise your arms overhead.

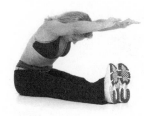

B

Reach your arms out from your shoulders. Exhale as you bend forward and reach for your toes. Hold 15 seconds. Release.

1-MINUTE EASY FIDGETSIZERS

Copy this page and carry it with you to remind yourself of your fidgetsizer options. For complete information on each exercise, see page 97.

Denise's Energizing Standing Roll-Down and Roll-Up

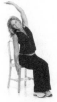

Side Bend

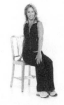

Seated Twist

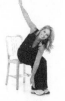

Seated Forward Bend

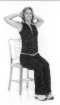

Seated Back Bend

10-MINUTE CORE COMPLETE ROUTINE FOR JUMP-START PHASE

Use this convenient at-a-glance page to complete your jump-start routine. For full details on each exercise, see page 112.

Seated Side Stretch

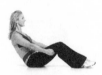
Pilates Beginner Roll-Up

Lower-Tummy Firmer

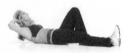
Straight-Leg Crunch I

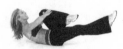
Pilates Single-Leg Stretch

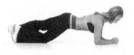
Low Hover II

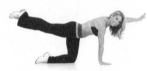
Back Strengthener I

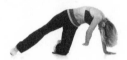
Pilates Beginner T-Stand

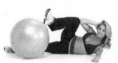
Side Crunch with Ball

Crunch on Ball

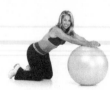
Roll-Out I

Torso Trimmer

Seated Chest Stretch

20-MINUTE CORE CARDIO BLAST FOR JUMP-START PHASE

Use this at-a-glance guide to complete your jump-start cardio blast. For complete details on each exercise, turn to page 126.

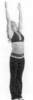

Warmup Standing Stretch

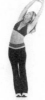

Warmup Standing Side Stretch

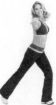

Front Jab

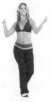

Mambo

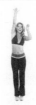

Basketball Shuffle

Squat with Shoulder Shaper

Lunge with Chest Fly I

Lunge with Side Chop

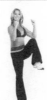

Triceps Toner

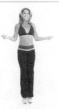

Jump Rope

Squat Knee Lift

Cha Cha

Plié Squat with Biceps Curl I

Deadlift into Double-Arm Row

Standing Pilates Swimming

(continued)

20-MINUTE CORE CARDIO BLAST
FOR JUMP-START PHASE *(cont.)*

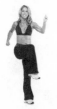

Marching in Place

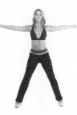

Jumping Jacks

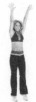

Knee Bend
with Overhead Reach

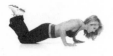

Pushup I

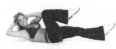

Pilates Crisscross I

Reverse Crunch

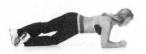

Plank I

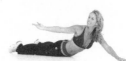

Swan

Butt Kick

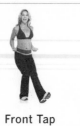

Front Tap

Leg Lift

Forward Bend

10-MINUTE CORE COMPLETE ROUTINE
FOR KEEP-ON-LOSING PHASE

Use this at-a-glance guide to help you follow your Keep-On-Losing routine. For full exercise details, turn to page 154.

Seated Side Stretch

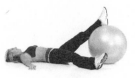

Heel Tap

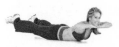

Lower-Tummy and Pelvic-Floor Strengthener on the Ball

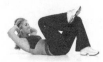

Straight-Leg Crunch II

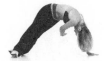

Pilates Full T-Stand

Back Strengthener II

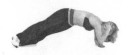

Waistline Slimmer

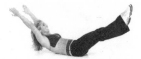

Pilates Double-Leg Stretch

Waistline Chop on the Ball

Tummy Tuck

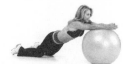

Roll-Out II

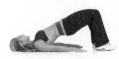

Yoga Bridge Stretch

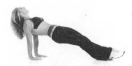

Reverse Plank Stretch

25-MINUTE CORE CARDIO BLAST
FOR KEEP-ON-LOSING PHASE

Use this at-a-glance guide to help you follow your Keep-On-Losing routine. For full exercise details, turn to page 168.

 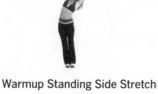

| Warmup Standing Stretch | Warmup Standing Side Stretch | Uppercuts |

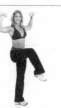 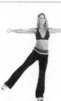 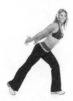

| Lunge with Chest Fly I | Side Lunge with Lateral Raise | Triceps Toner |

| Plié Squat with Biceps Curl II | Deadlift into Double-Arm Row | Standing Pilates Swimming |

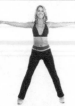

| Jumping Jacks | Pilates Crisscross II | Roll-Over |

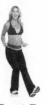 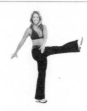 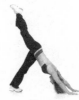

| Front Tap | Side Leg Kick | Plank into Down Dog |

Squat with Kick

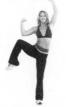

Abdominal Pull

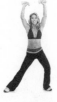

Side Lunge with
Overhead Press

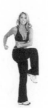

Jump Rope

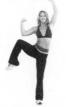

Knee-Up

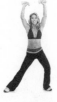

Lateral Bounding

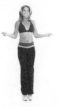

Pushup II

Side Kick

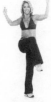

Side Twist

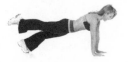

Plank II

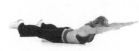

Superman

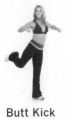

Butt Kick

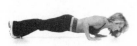

Forward Bend

PART FOUR

THE TUMMY TYPE PROGRAM

12 YOUR 2-WEEK JUMP-START PLANNER

Day-by-Day Meal Plans, Exercise Routines, Tips, and Inspiration to Motivate You toward Success

Welcome to the 2-week Jump-Start Phase of the Tone Your Tummy Type program! In this chapter, you will find 2 weeks of menus, exercise prescriptions, tips, and tools that will help you navigate this rapid-results phase of the plan one day at a time, in small, manageable baby steps. During this jump-start phase, you will notice dramatic results! The 1,300-daily-calorie meal plan will help your body to shed fat fast, while the gentle exercise prescriptions will enable you to slowly increase your fitness, even if you are a beginner.

On each of the next 14 days, you will find suggested meals to eat for breakfast, lunch, dinner, and a daily snack. You may eat your snack at any time of the day. Save it for when you—based on your lifestyle and hunger cues—most need it.

These meal suggestions come straight from the Core Diet recipes in Chapter 15. Don't let the "recipes" for breakfasts or snacks scare you. Quite often, these so-called recipes are as simple as spreading peanut butter on an apple or mixing fruit into a container of yogurt. I specifically designed them for busy people—just like you! On some days, your "recipe" is as simple as opening a frozen dinner and sticking it in the microwave or heading to your favorite Italian restaurant—how easy is that?

On appropriate days of the plan, you'll find reminders to complete various Core workouts. Remembering these routines is simple. Just turn to pages 195 to 201 to find a spread of thumbnail photos depicting each of these routines in sequence. You can rest the book on the floor or coffee table and periodically glance down to see what comes next in the routine. (For a detailed description of how to do each exercise, see Chapter 11.)

Now, I know your mother told you never to write in books—I know I've told my kids the same thing! But I encourage you to write in this planner—even if it's with a pencil. That way, you can refer to it later, when you are maintaining your weight loss. Place a star next to meals and snacks that you love. (Although I hope you love every single meal option, you might also cross out any meals or snacks that you don't enjoy or find too cumbersome to prepare.) Write notes in the margins to remind yourself how you felt or about the successes and challenges you face along the way. Later, you can look back over your notes to create a plan to keeping off the weight.

BEFORE YOU START

I encourage you to take a day or two to prepare your body, mind, and kitchen for the Tone Your Tummy Type program. Taking the extra steps I outline below will put you on the right path and ensure your success on this program.

Preparing Your Body

Practice the exercises outlined in "A Test Before You Start" on page 107 in Chapter 11. These exercises will help you to create the fitness foundation you need to correctly execute the 10-Minute Core Complete and 20-Minute Core Cardio Blast routines. Over the next few days, do the two simple moves first thing in the morning and once or twice again later in the day.

To get yourself psyched up and ready to go, prepare a place in your home to do your workouts. You don't need a lot of space. Most people find their living room works just fine. You'll need enough space to lie on the floor with your legs extended and arms extended either overhead or out to the sides. It's your little spot to target your tummy and slim your body.

Also, to complete the routines, you will need a set of light dumbbells and a fitness ball (sometimes called a stability ball or Swiss ball). Your dumbbells should be fairly light; 3 to 5 pounds will do. The fitness ball is an optional component to the plan. The few exercises that include it are super-effective, but if you do not have the means to purchase a ball, you can skip these exercises, doing extra repetitions of the other tummy movements instead.

Look for your dumbbells and fitness ball at any large sporting goods store, such as Sports Authority, and at most discount stores, such as Wal-Mart or Target. Consult the table below to figure out the best size ball for your body.

YOUR HEIGHT	BALL DIAMETER
4'11"–5'4"	53 cm (21")
5'5"–5'11"	65 cm (25")
6' and up	75 cm (29")

Sit on your ball as often as possible over the next few days. This will help you learn to engage your abs, because you'll have to use these muscles to keep yourself balanced. Consider using the ball as a desk chair. Sit on it while you supervise your child or children in the bath. Use it in the living room while you watch TV. Use your imagination. I even find it also makes a comfortable footrest.

Preparing Your Mind

You're about to embark on what may be a very different way of eating and way of moving your body. You're about to embark on a change. You may feel silly and even frustrated, for example, as you try new and unfamiliar exercises. Cooking new recipes—no matter how quick and easy their design—takes time.

So plan for it. Take a look at your schedule during the next 4 weeks and try to clear as many unnecessary stressors and time-consuming tasks off your schedule as possible. You might ask your spouse or kids to pitch in more around the house or ask a co-worker to help you with a big project. Make slimming down your midsection your number one priority for the next 4 weeks.

To create more time for this important life change, you may even consider scaling back on social commitments. That may mean skipping your book group or a volunteer activity this month. You don't have to give everything up, but you do need to be realistic. If you're the type of person who eats out every single night, you'll need to create some time in your day to try new recipes. If you've never exercised before, you'll need to find roughly 20 minutes a day for that pursuit. This time must come from somewhere—and, for most people, that means something else must drop off the to-do list. It's often easiest to find that time if you wake up a half hour earlier to fit it in your routine.

In addition to taking a good, hard look at your calendar, I recommend you take your measurements (especially your waist measurement), weigh yourself, and snap a photo of yourself. Use these measurements to motivate yourself toward your goal. Although your weight will fluctuate from day to day, a weekly weigh-in—as I recommend in this plan—will help you to see the success of your new eating and exercise habits. Consider taking a photo of yourself once a week while on this program and placing the photos next to each other on your fridge so that you can see your success every time you open the refrigerator door.

Preparing Your Kitchen

For the next 4 weeks, you will eat very little saturated fats, trans fats, added sugars, and starchy carbohydrates. To remove temptation, I want you to go through your kitchen cabinets and remove and toss (or donate to a food kitchen) the following items.

* Dairy products made from whole milk, including ice cream
* Fatty cuts of beef and other meats (including dark-meat chicken and any beef that is not called sirloin, tenderloin, or ground sirloin)

* Refined snack foods made from white flour (this describes any snack food that does not claim it's "100 percent whole grain" on the label)
* White bread
* White rice
* Fried foods (including frozen dinners that contain fried foods)

Once you've completed your "cleanup," it's time to head to the grocery store. Your first grocery shopping session may take you longer than usual, as you'll be hunting down some unfamiliar foods. It may also cost more than usual. Don't let your bill scare you! Many of the items on your week 1 shopping list will carry you through the 4-week meal plan—and beyond. As you progress on the plan, you'll see that each week's shopping list becomes progressively shorter—and your checkout bill much less expensive as a result.

On the following list, I've included a Greek yogurt as well as Stonyfield Farm yogurt. When I'm watching my weight, I like to choose the fat-free Greek yogurt because I get a nice, filling snack that's rich in protein for just a few calories, and I like to add a teaspoon of my favorite jam or honey. Other times I want to make sure I'm getting enough calcium, so I'll choose the calcium-rich Stonyfield Farm brand. If you can't find this brand, substitute a fat-free yogurt that contains roughly 80 calories and 300 milligrams of calcium per 6-ounce serving.

When using the following shopping list, feel free to substitute ingredients such as soy milk for cow's milk, tofu crumbles for ground turkey, or soy cheese for mozzarella. Simply follow the calorie and nutrient guidelines provided in the grocery list. If your substitution matches the nutrients mentioned, go for it! If you're not buying fresh meat or fish as you need it, keep it frozen until you're ready to use it and defrost just what you need. You can also store shredded feta and string cheese in the freezer. Keep the cheese in the original packaging and place that packaging inside a zipper-lock bag to ensure freshness. Take it out and let it thaw on the counter when you're ready to get started with your meal, then return the cheese to the freezer.

I've organized the following list into the basic categories you'll find at the store.

Week 1 Shopping List

Produce

2 cups fresh baby spinach leaves

1 (16-ounce) bag baby carrots

2 ounces grapes, red or green

12 ounces tofu, any type (firm, silken, etc.) with calcium sulfate listed as an ingredient*

2 cucumbers

1 orange

1 (2-ounce) brown potato

3 medium apples

4 tomatoes, small size such as Roma variety

2 medium yellow or white onions

2 green bell peppers

½ cup mushrooms†

2 kiwifruit

1 cup cherries†

1 cup strawberries†

½ cup raspberries†

2 mangoes

4 cloves garlic (1 small bunch) or 1 medium jar minced garlic*

2 tablespoons lemon juice (or the juice from 1 fresh lemon) or 1 small bottle lemon juice*

2 cups romaine lettuce

2 cups cole slaw greens (look for prewashed, precut bag)

1 nectarine

2 cups broccoli†

1 small box raisins* (1½ ounces)

Dairy

4 (6-ounce) containers fat-free plain yogurt with 80 calories and at least 300 milligrams calcium such as Stonyfield Farm brand

3 (6-ounce) containers fat-free plain Greek yogurt with 80 calories

1 (6-ounce) container fat-free fruit-flavored yogurt with no more than 140 calories and at least 300 milligrams calcium, such as Stonyfield Farm brand

1 (6-ounce) container fat-free lemon yogurt with no more than 140 calories and at least 300 milligrams calcium, such as Stonyfield Farm Lotsa Lemon

1 (10-ounce) container fat-free sour cream

1 (8-ounce) container calcium-fortified orange juice

2 dozen eggs* (separate and use egg whites only) or 3 (8-ounce) cartons egg substitute*

½ gallon fat-free milk

8 ounces reduced-fat feta cheese*

1 (8-ounce) package reduced-fat shredded Cheddar cheese such as Sargento Light 33% Reduced Fat*

3 (8-ounce) packages reduced-fat shredded mozzarella cheese such as Sargento Light 33% Reduced Fat*

½ ounce soft goat cheese

4 ounces tahini butter or tahini spread*

8 ounces hummus*

24 ounces (or 3 cups) 1% or fat-free cottage cheese (for weeks 1 and 2)

1 (8-ounce) container grated Parmesan cheese*

12 whole wheat soft tortillas (8" size), about 120 calories and at least 3 grams fiber per tortilla* (freeze)

1 package (4 sticks) light string cheese (look for 70 calories and less than 2 grams saturated fat per stick*)

24 ounces (or 3 cups) fat-free ricotta cheese*

Canned Foods

1 (12-ounce) can chunk light tuna packed in water

1 (8-ounce) can cannellini beans or white kidney beans

1 small jar unsweetened applesauce

1 (8-ounce) can unsweetened apple juice

*This amount will last through the entire 4-week plan.
†Choose either fresh or unsweetened, plain frozen variety.

1 (16-ounce) can chickpeas, also known as garbanzo or ceci beans

1 (8-ounce) can pinto beans

1 (8-ounce) can vegetarian beans

1 (8-ounce) can tomato soup such as Campbell's Low-Sodium Tomato Soup with Tomato Pieces or Healthy Choice Creamy Tomato Soup

1 (16-ounce) can Campbell's Healthy Request Minestrone Soup

1 (8-ounce) can no-salt-added chopped tomatoes

1 (16-ounce) can kidney beans

1 (8-ounce) can black beans

1 (16-ounce) can low-sodium chicken broth

1 (8-ounce) can fat-free refried beans

1 small jar or can artichoke hearts packed in water (about 10 artichoke hearts)

1 (8-ounce) can great Northern beans

1 (16-ounce) can beef vegetable soup such as Campbell's Healthy Request Beef Vegetable or Progresso 99% Fat-Free Beef Vegetable Soup

1 (16-ounce) can cream of mushroom soup such as Campbell's Healthy Request Cream of Mushroom Soup

1 (16-ounce) can lentil soup such as Health Valley Fat Free Lentil and Carrot Soup or Progresso 99% Fat-Free Lentil Soup

1 (8-ounce) can water chestnuts packed in water

Bread

1 package of 6 whole wheat English muffins (look for 130 calories and at least 3 grams fiber per muffin)

1 loaf whole wheat bread (look for 80 calories and at least 3 grams fiber per slice)

1 package of 8 whole wheat pitas (look for 160 calories and at least 3 grams fiber per pita)

1 small loaf whole grain rye bread (look for 80 calories and at least 2 grams fiber per slice)

1 small loaf whole grain pumpernickel bread

(look for 80 calories and at least 2 grams fiber per slice)

1 package of 6 whole wheat rolls (look for 160 calories and about 3 grams fiber per roll)

3 Boboli Whole Wheat Thin Pizza Crusts (12" size)

Cereals/Pasta

1 small box whole wheat couscous

1 (16-ounce) box or bag whole wheat pasta

1 (16-ounce) box brown rice

1 small box orzo

1 small box quinoa

1 small jar wheat germ

1 (20-ounce) or smallest-size box low-fat granola such as Healthy Choice brand (without raisins)

1 (20-ounce) or smallest-size box Kashi Good Friends or Cheerios cereal

1 (20-ounce) or smallest-size box Kashi Heart to Heart or Barbara's Bakery Grainshop cereal

1 (18-ounce) canister quick-cooking oatmeal

1 small box instant packets of grits

1 box Kellogg's All-Bran Breakfast Bar (any flavor)

1 (20-ounce) or smallest-size box muesli such as Healthy Choice brand

Crackers/Snacks

1 Weight Watchers Fat-Free Blueberry Muffin (or 170 calories' worth of muffin)

1 Weight Watchers Honey-Roasted Peanuts

1 box 94% reduced-fat microwave popcorn

1 bag (3 ounces for all 6 weeks) baked tortilla chips (any variety)

1 small box plain graham crackers

1 box Ak-Mak crackers or Reduced-Fat Triscuit Crackers or any cracker with no trans fats and at least 3 grams fiber per serving

Nuts/Baking/Spices

1 small bag pine nuts/pignolas

1 large bag (2 cups) slivered almonds

1 small jar dry-roasted unsalted peanuts

1 small bag (1 cup) chopped pecans

1 small bag (½ cup) roasted unsalted soy nuts

1 small bag (¾ cup) chopped walnuts

1 small bag (10 nuts) walnut halves

1 small can nonstick spray

1 small can olive oil–flavored nonstick spray

1 small can butter-flavored nonstick spray

1 small bottle white vinegar

1 small bottle rice vinegar

1 small bottle red wine vinegar

1 small bottle balsamic vinegar

1 small bag whole wheat pastry flour

1 small box dehydrated potato flakes

1 small jar sesame seeds

1 small bottle pure vanilla extract

1 small jar poppy seeds

1 small bottle white cooking wine

1 small bottle red cooking wine

1 small bottle cooking sherry

1 small bag (¼ cup) sunflower seeds

1 small bottle sesame oil

1 bottle (9 ounces or more) extra-virgin olive oil

1 small bottle sunflower oil

1 small bottle canola oil

1 small bag flax meal

1 small box whole wheat pancake mix

1 small box brown sugar

1 small jar ground cinnamon

1 small jar paprika

1 small ground black pepper

1 small jar dried dill

1 small jar dried basil

1 small jar ground nutmeg

1 small jar dried sage

1 small jar dried parsley

1 small jar dried rosemary

1 small jar dried thyme

1 small jar dried oregano

1 small jar dried chives

1 small jar onion powder

1 small jar caraway seeds

1 small jar ground ginger

1 small jar ground oregano

1 small jar chili powder

1 small jar ground cumin

1 small jar dill seed

1 small jar curry powder

1 small jar garlic powder

1 small jar capers (if desired)

1 small jar Old Bay seasoning

Condiments/Sauces

1 small bottle Worcestershire sauce

1 small bottle barbecue sauce

1 small jar honey

1 small jar cocktail sauce

1 (16-ounce) jar spaghetti sauce, less than 350 milligrams sodium per ½-cup serving

1 small jar black olives

1 small jar Dijon mustard

1 small bottle reduced-sodium teriyaki sauce

1 small bottle reduced-sodium soy sauce

1 small jar apricot jam

1 small jar natural peanut butter

1 small jar almond butter

1 small jar roasted red peppers

1 (24-ounce) jar salsa

1 small bottle light Caesar salad dressing

1 small bottle light ranch salad dressing

1 small bottle fat-free creamy Italian salad dressing

1 small bottle light salad dressing (your choice if you need more variety than ranch or Caesar)

1 small bottle maple syrup

1 small bottle canola oil light mayonnaise

1 small box prepared falafel mix such as Fantastic Foods brand

1 small canister seasoned bread crumbs

1 small box cornbread mix

Meat/Seafood

1 (6-ounce) piece halibut, sole, or flounder

1 (4-ounce) piece orange roughy

1 (4-ounce) piece salmon steak

2 (4-ounce) and 1 (5-ounce) boneless, skinless chicken breasts (13 ounces total) (weeks 1 and 2)

1 (4-ounce) piece beef tenderloin

6 ounces ground turkey breast (weeks 1 and 2)

Deli

9 ounces sliced deli chicken breast

2½ ounces Jarlsberg Lite or Alpine Lace 50% reduced-fat Swiss cheese

10 ounces sliced ham such as Applegate Farms No Nitrites Added Uncured Ham

3 ounces sliced turkey breast

3 ounces sliced lean roast beef such as Healthy Choice brand

Frozen Ready-Made Meals

1 Weight Watchers Smart Ones English Muffin Sandwich

1 Morningstar Farms Breakfast Sandwich with Cheese

1 Amy's Kitchen Indian Mattar Tofu

1 Healthy Choice Manicotti with Three Cheeses

1 Amy's Kitchen Country Cheddar Bowl

1 Amy's Kitchen Vegetable Lasagna

1 Healthy Choice Grilled Whiskey Steak

1 Amy's Kitchen Stuffed Pasta Shells Bowl

1 Weight Watchers Smart Ones Salisbury Steak

Other Frozen

1 box of 6-count low-fat whole grain waffles with 170 calories and at least 6 grams of fiber per 2-waffle serving, such as Kashi Good Friends

1 (16-ounce) bag cut-leaf spinach

1 (16-ounce) package white or yellow corn

1 package of veggie sausage patties such as Morningstar Farms Breakfast Patties (or look for 80 calories and 3 grams fat or less per patty)

1 (16-ounce) bag Chinese style vegetables (includes bok choy, broccoli, carrots, or water chestnuts)

1 small Boca Meatless Chick'n Nuggets or Tyson Low-Fat Chicken Patty

1 small bag peas

Other/Checkout Aisle

20 chocolate-covered espresso beans

1 Pria Bar

READY, SET, GO!

Now that you've done your homework—you've prepared your body, mind, and kitchen—you're ready to get started. The following pages will take you step by step through phase 1 of the plan. Once you've completed it, you can move on to phase 2. You'll find everything you need to know about phase 2 in Chapters 13 and 14. Good luck!

 DAY 1

DENISE'S DAILY WISDOM

If your tummy could talk, it would tell you that it doesn't like to sit! When you sit, you tend to slouch, which allows your tummy to sag outward. When you stand, you must firm your tummy muscles to support your body weight. Plus, standing burns more calories than sitting. So sort the mail while standing up. Talk on the phone while standing (or, better yet, while walking).

TODAY'S WORKOUT

Core Complete routine (see pages 112 to 125) plus 20 minutes of cardio of your choice

HOW TO TELL IF A PRODUCT IS WHOLE GRAIN

When shopping for whole grain products, look for any of the following whole grains as the *first ingredient listed*, and follow the guidelines outlined in the grocery list for calories and grams of fiber as well.

- ☐ Whole wheat
- ☐ Whole oats
- ☐ Brown rice

- ☐ Bulgur
- ☐ Graham flour
- ☐ Oatmeal

- ☐ Whole grain corn
- ☐ Whole rye
- ☐ Wild rice

TODAY'S MENU

Breakfast

Tone Your Tummy Type On-the-Go Muffin (page 259)

6 ounces fat-free plain Greek yogurt topped with ¼ cup sliced frozen grapes (freeze for at least 1 hour)

Lunch

Asian Chicken with Couscous (page 260)

Snack

2 tablespoons soy nuts

1 stick light string cheese

1 cup fat-free milk

Dinner

Orange-Glazed Salmon with Pecans (page 260)

Nutrition Analysis

1,314 calories, 107 g protein (32%), 131 g carbohydrates (40%), 40 g total fat (28%), 9 g saturated fat (6%), 167 mg cholesterol, 21 g dietary fiber, 2,001 mg sodium, 985 mg calcium

---

FUN TUMMY TRUTH

The same plaque that causes gum disease in your mouth can trigger inflammation throughout your body, raising your risk of heart disease and causing you to store tummy fat.

DAY 2

DENISE'S DAILY WISDOM

The next time you feel like driving to the local coffee shop for a latte pick-me-up, try this simple breathing technique instead. It will give you an instant burst of energy while you simultaneously tone your tummy. Called the breath of fire, this yoga breathing technique can be done by inhaling deeply and then exhaling 20 to 30 short, rapid bursts of air, pumping out the air with your tummy muscles. As your tummy pumps inward, it forces the air outward. This technique squeezes out every last bit of stale carbon dioxide in your lungs, helping to fully oxygenate your body, giving you a nice burst of energy.

TODAY'S WORKOUT

Core Cardio Blast routine (see pages 126 to 153)

TODAY'S MENU

Breakfast
6 ounces Stonyfield Farm Lotsa Lemon yogurt combined with ½ cup Kashi Heart to Heart cereal (or 1 cup Barbara's Bakery GrainShop cereal) and 1 tablespoon slivered almonds

Lunch
Pinto Bean Bowl (page 261)

1 apple

Snack
1 cup 1% fat or fat-free cottage cheese mixed with 2 tablespoons low-fat granola cereal

Dinner
Parmesan Turkey Pasta with Vegetables (page 261)

Nutrition Analysis
1,290 calories, 95 g protein (29%), 179 g carbohydrates (55%), 28 g total fat (20%), 5 g saturated fat (3%), 48 mg cholesterol, 34 g dietary fiber, 2,168 mg sodium, 890 mg calcium

---

FUN TUMMY TRUTH
Your stomach has to produce a new layer of mucus every 2 weeks to prevent its gastric juices from digesting itself.

The Tummy Type Program

DENISE'S DAILY WISDOM

If you experience a lot of bloating in your tummy from gastrointestinal distress or around your period, try using the following Chinese Medicine technique. I find that it helps to get a sluggish digestive tract moving. To do it, lie on your back. Place your right palm on your stomach, just above your navel. Place your left palm on top of the right. Use your hands to rub your tummy 20 to 40 times gently in a clockwise motion. Then place your palms just below either side of your rib cage and massage downward toward your groin 5 times.

TODAY'S WORKOUT

A 20-minute power walk

TODAY'S MENU

Breakfast
Cherry Smoothie (page 261)

Lunch
Poppy Chicken Salad (page 262)

Snack
1 sliced mango with 1½ slices of Alpine Lace reduced-fat Swiss cheese or Jarlsberg Lite Swiss cheese

Dinner
Pasta with Chickpeas (page 262)

Nutrition Analysis
1,327 calories, 68 g protein (20%), 189 g carbohydrates (56%), 40 g total fat (27%), 9 g saturated fat (6%), 78 mg cholesterol, 31 g dietary fiber, 1,172 mg sodium, 1,224 mg calcium

---

FUN TUMMY TRUTH
Although it takes roughly 30 seconds to chew your food and 10 seconds to swallow it, it takes nearly 3 to 4 hours for the gastric juices in your stomach to break it down and another 18 to 48 hours for it to move through your intestine!

DAY 4

DENISE'S DAILY WISDOM

Keep a dozen hard-cooked eggs in the fridge at all times. Just boil them up and either place them back in the egg carton or store them in a zipper-lock bag. Then you'll always have some lean protein ready when you need it for a quick snack or to top a salad. To reduce the number of calories eggs usually provide, I like to eat half of the yolk. I feed the other half to my dog, who considers it a wonderful treat.

TODAY'S WORKOUT

Core Complete routine (see pages 112 to 125) plus 20 minutes of cardio of your choice

TODAY'S MENU

Breakfast
Maple Ricotta Cereal Bowl (page 262)

Lunch
Pita Triangles and Bean Dip (page 263)

Snack
1 Tone Your Tummy Type On-the-Go Muffin

6 ounces fat-free Greek yogurt

Dinner
Mild Cajun Fish Stew (page 263)

Nutrition Analysis
1,353 calories, 89 g protein (28%), 180 g carbohydrates (52%), 35 g total fat (22%), 4 g saturated fat (3%), 100 mg cholesterol, 28 g dietary fiber, 1,401 mg sodium, 925 mg calcium

---

FUN TUMMY TRUTH
Laugh hard. Not only does it feel great and blast away stress, it firms your tummy muscles, especially if you have a good "belly" laugh.

The Tummy Type Program

DAY 5

DENISE'S DAILY WISDOM

Today you will eat out for the first time on the plan. I bet you didn't think you'd be able to eat spaghetti and meatballs and still shrink tummy fat! To eat out successfully, however, you must pay careful attention to your portions. Most Italian restaurants serve up much more than 1 cup of pasta with your meal. To keep yourself from eating "just a little bit more" after you know you've had your fill, ask your waiter to serve up only the recommended amount, putting the rest in a take-out container before it reaches the table or share it with your honey or friend.

TODAY'S WORKOUT

Core Cardio Blast routine (see pages 126 to 153)

TODAY'S MENU

Breakfast
Apple, Potato, and Egg Skillet (page 264)

Lunch
Honey and Garlic Chicken with Brown Rice (page 264)

Snack
Cucumber with Creamy Tahini Spread (page 264)

Dinner
Eat out at your favorite Italian restaurant! Order the house salad (no cheese) and top with 1 tablespoon salad dressing or a little vinegar plus 1 teaspoon extra-virgin olive oil. Have spaghetti with meat sauce or meatballs for your main course. Make sure to stop at just 1 cup pasta with ½ cup meat sauce or ⅓ cup marinara sauce with 2 meatballs (1½" diameter), each about the size of a ping-pong ball.

Nutrition Analysis
1,295 calories, 73 g protein (23%), 186 g carbohydrates (57%), 34 g total fat (23%), 9 g saturated fat (6%), 71 mg cholesterol, 21 g dietary fiber, 1,969 mg sodium, 1,032 mg calcium

---

FUN TUMMY TRUTH
A person swallows about 295 times while eating dinner.

DAY 6

DENISE'S DAILY WISDOM

Tonight you'll eat lean beef for dinner. When shopping for beef, look for a grass-fed variety. These days, most conventional beef comes from cows that eat grains from a feedlot. Cows that graze on grass, however, tend to produce beef that contains more of a healthful type of fat called conjugated linoleic acid (CLA). In one study, people who consumed 4 grams of CLA a day lost 4 percent body fat—mostly in the tummy area—over 12 weeks, even though they made no other lifestyle changes. Eating grass-fed beef and poultry is one way to ensure you get enough CLA in your diet.

TODAY'S WORKOUT

Day off—but have some active fun!

TODAY'S MENU

Breakfast

1 Tone Your Tummy Type On-the-Go Muffin

6 ounces fat-free Greek yogurt topped with ½ cup raspberries

Lunch

Hummus and Baked Chips (page 265)

Snack

Bell Pepper and Carrots with Onion Dip (page 265)

Dinner

Beef Tenderloin and Mediterranean Spinach (page 265)

Nutrition Analysis

1,340 calories, 82 g protein (25%), 164 g carbohydrates (49%), 40 g total fat (27%), 10 g saturated fat (7%), 110 mg cholesterol, 29 g dietary fiber, 1,726 mg sodium, 916 mg calcium

---

FUN TUMMY TRUTH

A toothpick is the object most often choked on by Americans.

DENISE'S DAILY WISDOM

If you have a dog, walk it rather than simply letting it out the door to do its business. When the Institute for National Resources in Concord, California, calculated the caloric expenditures for typical activities, it determined that walking a dog for 30 minutes burns 125 calories; letting the dog out the back door and then resting on the couch burns 2. Dogs make great walking companions, ones who will poke and prod you into getting outdoors, no matter the weather.

ASSESS YOUR SUCCESS

Take your measurements or step on the scale. Take another photo of yourself. How much weight have you lost? How many inches have you lost in your waistline?

TAKE TIME TO REFLECT

What went well for you last week, and what did not go so well? Did you follow the meal plan without fail, or did you stray from time to time? If you cheated, what caused you to stray? Similarly, if you skipped any of the suggested workouts, what caused you to backslide? To help solidify your resolve to improve during week 2, take a good, hard look at the reasons behind why you did or did not follow the plan.

TODAY'S WORKOUT

Day off—rest, rejuvenate, and relax

TODAY'S MENU

Breakfast
Strawberry Smoothie: In a blender, combine 1 cup fresh or unsweetened, frozen strawberries; 3 tablespoons calcium-fortified orange juice; 3 ounces firm tofu (made with calcium sulfate); 1 tablespoon wheat germ; and 1 cup fat-free milk.

Lunch
Chicken Pita (page 266)

Snack

1 Kellogg's All-Bran Breakfast Bar spread with 2 teaspoons peanut butter

Dinner

At your favorite create-your-own burrito restaurant, start your burrito with the 12" tortilla wrap, add ½ cup black beans, 1 cup fajita-style vegetables, lettuce, tomato and ¼ cup guacamole. If you prefer to eat at home, heat up a frozen vegetarian burrito (such as Don Miguel Lean Olé! varieties or Del Taco Veggie Works). If you choose a frozen burrito, serve with 1 banana on the side.

Nutrition Analysis

1,299 calories, 80 g protein (25%), 162 g carbohydrates (49%), 30 g total fat (21%), 7 g saturated fat (5%), 85 mg cholesterol, 58 g dietary fiber, 2,462 mg sodium, 993 mg calcium

FUN TUMMY TRUTH

Acupuncturists believe you can press a point on the head to control your appetite. It is located in the hollow just in front of the flap of the ear.

Week 2 Shopping List

Produce

4 baby zucchini*

3 apricots

1 peach

1 banana

1 orange

1 papaya

1 medium apple

7 tomatoes, small size such as Roma variety

1 red bell pepper

1 medium yellow or white onion

1 green bell pepper

1½ cups mushrooms†

½ cup blueberries†

¾ cup strawberries†

5 slices soy cheese, 40 calories and 2 grams of fat, and less than 1 gram saturated fat per slice*

½ cup blackberries†

1 rib celery

2 tablespoons lemon juice or the juice from 1 fresh lemon

2 cups arugula

2 cups romaine lettuce

2 cups coleslaw greens (look for prewashed, precut bag)

1 scallion or green onion

1 cup broccoli†

1 cup cauliflower†

1 small eggplant

1 ear of corn, yellow or white

Dairy

1 (6-ounce) container fat-free vanilla yogurt with 140 calories or less and at least 300 milligrams calcium, such as Stonyfield Farm French Vanilla

2 (6-ounce) containers fat-free plain yogurt with 80 calories and at least 300 milligrams calcium, such as Stonyfield Farm brand

1 (6-ounce) container fat-free plain Greek yogurt with 80 calories

1 (6-ounce) container fat-free fruit-flavored yogurt with 140 calories or less and at least 300 milligrams calcium, such as Stonyfield Farm Peach, Raspberry, Strawberry, French Vanilla, Apricot Mango, Berry Bash, Black Cherry, or Blueberry

1 (8-ounce) tub light butter with canola oil, such as Land O'Lakes brand*

1 quart (or 32 ounces) fat-free milk

Meat/Seafood

1 (4-ounce) piece orange roughy

1 (7-ounce) piece salmon steak

Deli

3 ounces sliced turkey breast

3 ounces sliced lean roast beef, such as Healthy Choice brand

*This amount will last through the entire 4-week plan.
†Choose either fresh or unsweetened, plain frozen variety.

DAY 8

DENISE'S DAILY WISDOM

As I've mentioned before, stress raises levels of the hormone cortisol, which triggers fat storage in your abdomen. Stretching helps to relieve stress by soothing away muscle tension. Muscle tension and stress are closely interlinked. Reduce one and you tend to affect the other. So, whenever you are feeling tense, take a 5-minute break to stretch your body. You'll feel great afterward!

TODAY'S WORKOUT

Core Complete routine (see pages 112 to 125) plus 20 minutes of cardio of your choice

TODAY'S MENU

Breakfast

Tortilla with Sunflower Cucumber Spread (page 266)

Lunch

London Broil Chicken with Pesto (page 266)

Snack

Broccoli and Cauliflower with Onion Dip: Serve ½ of the onion dip left over from Day 6 with 1 cup each broccoli and cauliflower florets.

Dinner

Crunchy Salmon Cakes (page 267)

Nutrition Analysis

1,315 calories, 94 g protein (29%), 151 g carbohydrates (46%), 39 g total fat (27%), 9 g saturated fat (6%), 134 mg cholesterol, 27 g dietary fiber, 1,875 mg sodium, 1,139 mg calcium

---

FUN TUMMY TRUTH
After overeating, your hearing is less sharp.

DAY 9

DENISE'S DAILY WISDOM

Poor posture makes your tummy "pooch out." It accentuates skin rolls and allows everything to sag outward. Plus, it's bad for your back! So, periodically throughout the day, do a posture check. Stand tall, pressing into the floor as you lengthen your body upward. Relax your shoulders down, away from your ears. Bring your chin down and in as the top of your head rises. Then zip up those abs like a corset. Look how flat your tummy is!

TODAY'S WORKOUT

Core Cardio Blast routine (see pages 126 to 153)

TODAY'S MENU

Breakfast

Half of a Peanut Butter and Apricot Sandwich: Toast 1 slice of whole wheat bread, spread with 2 teaspoons peanut butter, and top with 1 sliced apricot. Slice, sharing the other half with one of your kids or your spouse.

6 ounces fat-free Greek yogurt

Lunch

Black Bean Roll-Up: Fill an 8" whole wheat soft tortilla with ½ cup cooked corn, ¼ cup canned black beans (rinsed and drained), ¼ cup salsa, and 2 tablespoons reduced-fat shredded Cheddar cheese.

1 cup fat-free milk

Snack

1 Tone Your Tummy Type On-the-Go Muffin spread with ¼ cup fat-free ricotta cheese mixed with 2 teaspoons maple syrup

Dinner

Salmon and Veggies with Spicy Ranch Sauce (page 267)

Nutrition Analysis

1,338 calories, 79 g protein (23%), 176 g carbohydrates (52%), 37 g total fat (25%), 9 g saturated fat (6%), 89 mg cholesterol, 40 g dietary fiber, 3,046 mg sodium, 1,006 mg calcium

FUN TUMMY TRUTH

Americans eat 134 pounds of sugar a year.

DENISE'S DAILY WISDOM

Dry, flaky skin on your tummy can accentuate the appearance of fat and saggy skin. To keep my skin healthy and supple—especially before a photo shoot—I like to massage Keri lotion into my abdomen after my morning shower. I use the lotion all over my body to hydrate my skin from head to toe, but I think it's important not to forget your tummy. When I mention this tip to my friends, I'm surprised by how many of them skip over their tummies when moisturizing their skin. They remember their arms and legs but neglect this important body area!

TODAY'S WORKOUT

A 20-minute power walk

TODAY'S MENU

Breakfast

Grilled Mushrooms, Tomato, and Mozzarella on Pumpernickel (page 267)

Lunch

Cabbage-Apple Salad (page 268)

Snack

1 whole-grain waffle such as Kashi Go Lean, toasted and topped with ½ cup blueberries

1 soy sausage patty (with about 80 calories, such as Morningstar Farms brand)

Dinner

Ratatouille (page 268)

Nutrition Analysis

1,279 calories, 77 g protein (24%), 182 g carbohydrates (54%), 35 g total fat (25%), 9 g saturated fat (6%), 35 mg cholesterol, 31 g dietary fiber, 2,094 mg sodium, 1,296 mg calcium

---

FUN TUMMY TRUTH

Americans eat 18 billion hot dogs a year.

DAY 11

DENISE'S DAILY WISDOM

The next time you find yourself running errands, make it your goal to get out of the car. So much of the world is now designed to make driving convenient. With drive-thru banks, liquor stores, pharmacies, and even coffee shops, you can run many errands without ever actually getting out of your car. Yet, when the Institute for National Resources in Concord, California, calculated the caloric expenditures for typical activities, they determined that parking a car and going into a store three times a week burns 70 calories, whereas sitting in your car at drive-thru windows burns only 15! So always get out and walk.

TODAY'S WORKOUT

Core Complete routine (see pages 112 to 125) plus 20 minutes of cardio of your choice

TODAY'S MENU

Breakfast

At your bagel shop, order ½ of a whole wheat, granola, or cinnamon-raisin bagel, topped with 1 tablespoon light veggie cream cheese, lettuce, tomato, and onion. Cut in half. Indulge with 1 tall (12-ounce) fat-free latte.

Lunch

Philadelphia Beef (page 268)

Snack

Honey Cream Oats: Combine ½ cup fat-free ricotta cheese with 1 teaspoon brown sugar and 1 teaspoon honey. Make oatmeal with 1 packet instant or ½ cup plain oatmeal. Mix oatmeal together with the ricotta cheese in a bowl.

Dinner

Orange Roughy and Arugula Blackberry Salad (page 269)

Nutrition Analysis

1,303 calories, 85 g protein (26%), 165 g carbohydrates (50%), 39 g total fat (27%), 11 g saturated fat (8%), 116 mg cholesterol, 21 g dietary fiber, 2,912 mg sodium, 1,483 mg calcium

---

FUN TUMMY TRUTH

Technically, a tummy tuck is called an abdominoplasty.

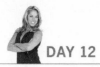

DAY 12

DENISE'S DAILY WISDOM

I must bare my tummy for many photo shoots and for filming my exercise shows and DVDs. Because of this, I take care when choosing the outfits I wear on the set. Over the years, I've noticed that tight waistbands can press tummy fat and skin upward, creating a visible roll of fat that otherwise would not be noticeable. So, look for clothes that aren't too tight around the middle. I like comfortable clothing that moves with me but does not press into my tummy, causing my skin to bunch up.

TODAY'S WORKOUT

Core Cardio Blast routine (see pages 126 to 153)

TODAY'S DAILY MENU

Breakfast

1 whole grain waffle such as Kashi Go Lean, toasted and topped with 6 ounces fat-free Stonyfield Farm French Vanilla yogurt and ¾ cup fresh or frozen, unsweetened strawberries

Lunch

Turkey Tahini Sandwich: Toast 1 whole wheat English muffin, spread with 2 tablespoons tahini butter, and fill with ¼ cup sliced red pepper and 3 ounces sliced turkey breast.

Snack

Cheesy Toast: Heat 1 slice pumpernickel bread topped with 2 slices soy cheese in a 200°F oven for about 2 to 3 minutes, or until the cheese is slightly melted.

1 orange

Dinner

Chili Soup (page 269)

Nutrition Analysis

1,285 calories, 74 g protein (23%), 192 g carbohydrates (57%), 30 g total fat (21%), 5 g saturated fat (4%), 50 mg cholesterol, 42 g dietary fiber, 2,706 mg sodium, 1,302 mg calcium

---

FUN TUMMY TRUTH

In addition to preventing urinary tract infections, cranberry juice may keep you from getting the stomach flu, researchers find.

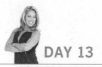

DAY 13

DENISE'S DAILY WISDOM

All of us have busy days when we just can't fit in an official workout. These types of days even happen to me—and this is my business. When I find myself in meetings, traveling, or running around with my kids and just can't squeeze in my workout no matter how hard I try (and I always try!), I do isometrics. I squeeze and release the muscles in my arms, legs, buns, back, and tummy over and over. The beauty of isometrics is that no one can tell you are doing them. So while sitting in a meeting, delivering a speech, or waiting at the ticket counter, start squeezing—especially "zipping up" your abs!

TODAY'S WORKOUT

Day off

TODAY'S MENU

Breakfast

Almond Butter Melt: In a bowl, heat 1 tablespoon almond butter in the microwave for 30 seconds. Add ½ cup cereal such as Kashi Good Friends or Cheerios or 60 calories of your favorite cereal and stir well to combine.

1 cup fat-free milk

Lunch

Taco Salad (page 270)

Snack

¾ cup 1% or fat-free cottage cheese mixed with 1 tablespoon apricot jam and ½ teaspoon vanilla extract and topped with 2 chopped fresh or canned (juice- or water-pack) apricots

Dinner

Tomato Couscous with Spicy Grilled Eggplant (page 270)

Nutrition Analysis

1,290 calories, 83 g protein (25%), 143 g carbohydrates (46%), 48 g total fat (32%), 13 g saturated fat (9%), 73 mg cholesterol, 27 g dietary fiber, 2,291 mg sodium, 919 mg calcium

FUN TUMMY TRUTH

Raspberries contain a phenol called ellagic tannin that inhibits the growth of harmful intestinal bacteria.

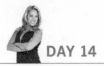

DENISE'S DAILY WISDOM

Egg whites are a great source of protein. Many of my recipes call for egg whites rather than the entire egg. Omitting the yolk saves you from eating saturated fat, cholesterol, and calories. Without the yolk, an entire egg has only 30 calories. If you (or your spouse or kids) don't like the look of white scrambled eggs or a white omelet, compromise by mixing in just one yolk. I've tried this with my family and find that it adds color and texture to egg dishes but only a minimum amount of fat and calories.

ASSESS YOUR SUCCESS

Take your measurements or step on the scale. Take another photo of yourself. How much weight have you lost? How many inches have you lost in your waistline?

TAKE TIME TO REFLECT

You've completed 2 weeks of the Tone Your Tummy Type program. Bravo! Be proud of yourself. You're doing great. Take a moment today to think about all of the things you did well during the past couple of weeks. Also, try to solve any problems. What changes can you make to increase your ability to exercise consistently to follow the menu plans?

TODAY'S WORKOUT

Day off—refresh and rejuvenate

TODAY'S MENU

Breakfast
Peach and Cottage Cheese Wrap (page 271)

Lunch
Grilled Vegetable Sandwich (page 271)

Snack
1 peeled banana sliced lengthwise and spread with 1 tablespoon peanut butter

Dinner
Dijon Chicken with Parmesan Vegetables (page 271)

Nutrition Analysis
1,336 calories, 73 g protein (22%), 171 g carbohydrates (51%), 46 g total fat (30%), 13 g saturated fat (9%), 117 mg cholesterol, 36 g dietary fiber, 1,214 mg sodium, 1,137 mg calcium

---

FUN TUMMY TRUTH

Your body weight may vary as much as 3 to 5 pounds a day, depending on your fluid balance and fluid retention.

PHASE 1 COMPLETE!

Congratulations for successfully completing the Jump-Start Phase. You've worked hard during the past 2 weeks, so give yourself a pat on the back for a job well done. Although you are now ready to move on to the Keep-On-Losing Phase of the plan, I encourage you to return to this jump-start plan whenever you find your tummy needs a tune-up. Getting ready for bikini season? Preparing for a high school reunion? Want to look fantastic at a wedding? This jump-start phase will get you the results you need.

I'm proud of you, and I hope you are equally proud of yourself. You've followed a new and healthy eating plan and started to make exercise an integral part of your life. You worked hard to learn new movements and new exercise routines. I know it's not always easy to follow the exercise routine laid out in a book—but I'm sure by now, you can see that it's worth it! You made the effort, and you succeeded!

Now you are ready to start the Keep-On-Losing Phase. You'll learn everything you need to know about it in Chapter 13, which provides information on phase 2 eating and exercising. Here, you'll find two new exercise routines. Based on the routines you completed during phase 1, your phase 2 routines include a few new moves as well as some variations on the moves you completed during phase 2.

So turn to the next chapter and continue your journey to a flatter, sexier tummy!

13 YOUR 2-WEEK KEEP-ON-LOSING-PHASE PLANNER

**You've Seen Dramatic Results.
Now Drop Even More Weight!**

Congratulations on your successful completion of the first 2 weeks of the Tone Your Tummy Type program! You've worked hard, so give yourself a pat on the back.

In the following pages you'll find everything you need to continue your journey toward success. Now you are ready to embark on the Keep-On-Losing Phase of the Tone Your Tummy Type program. During this phase, you will continue to lose weight, although at a pace that's more steady than you may have experienced during the Jump-Start Phase. This planner will guide you through your first 2 weeks of the Keep-On-Losing Phase, providing you with 2 weeks of menus, exercise prescriptions, tips, and tools.

In this phase, you will relax a little on your eating—allowing yourself 1,500 daily calories. As you follow the meal plan laid out in the following pages, you will continue to shed fat—and keep it off once you reach your goal. Your stepped-up exercise routine will help you to burn even more calories and fat than you did during phase 1. You'll also continue to shape and sculpt sexy, lean muscle throughout your body.

On each of the next 14 days, you will find suggested meals to eat for breakfast, lunch, dinner, and a daily snack. As with phase 1, you may eat your snack at any time of the day. Save it for when you—based on your lifestyle and hunger cues—most need it. These meal suggestions come straight from the phase 2 recipes in Chapter 15.

On appropriate days of the plan, you'll find reminders to complete various workouts. Turn to pages 199 to 201 to find a spread of thumbnail photos depicting each of these routines at a glance. For a detailed description of how to do each exercise, see Chapter 11.

As with phase 1, I encourage you to write in this planner.

Also, below you will find the ingredients you will need for the next week of the meal plan.

Week 3 Shopping List

Produce

3 cups baby spinach leaves

1 cup blueberries†

6 ounces grapes, red or green

1 banana

2 apples

5 tomatoes, small size such as Roma variety

1 red bell pepper

3 cups strawberries†

1 small red onion

1 mango

4 cups romaine lettuce

1 avocado

1 scallion

1 plum

Dairy

1 (6-ounce) container fat-free plain Greek yogurt with 80 calories

4 (6-ounce) containers fat-free fruit-flavored yogurt with 140 calories or less and at least 300 milligrams calcium, such as Stonyfield Farm Peach, Raspberry, Strawberry, French Vanilla, Apricot-Mango, Berry Bash, Black Cherry, or Blueberry

1 small flavored low-fat coffee creamer*

8 ounces fat-free sour cream

1 (8-ounce) tub light butter with canola oil, such as Land O'Lakes brand

½ gallon fat-free milk

3 ounces soft goat cheese*

1 package Laughing Cow cheese wedges (any flavor)

Meat/Seafood

1 (3-ounce) swordfish steak

4 ounces boneless, skinless chicken breast

*This amount will last through the rest of the 4-week plan.
†Choose either fresh or unsweetened, plain frozen variety.

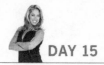

DAY 15

DENISE'S DAILY WISDOM

Remember to drink plenty of water. It's always important to stay hydrated, but especially important as you are losing weight and getting in better shape. You're losing more water through sweat during your workouts. You also need to keep your body well hydrated to burn fat. So do as I do and stash water bottles everywhere—in your purse, your car, your desk at work.

TODAY'S WORKOUT

Core Complete routine (see pages 154 to 167) plus 25 minutes of cardio of your choice

TODAY'S MENU

Breakfast

Cinnamon Apple Cereal: Chop 1 apple and mix with ¼ cup low-fat granola cereal, 4 teaspoons slivered almonds, ¼ teaspoon ground cinnamon, ½ cup fat-free milk. Heat in the microwave for 60 to 90 seconds.

Lunch

Creamy Spinach Pasta (page 272)

Snack

Tone Your Tummy Type On-the-Go Muffin

1 tall (12-ounce) fat-free milk latte

Dinner

Minestrone Soup and Bruschetta (page 272)

Nutrition Analysis

1,560 calories, 74 g protein (19%), 214 g carbohydrates (54%), 54 g total fat (31%), 10 g saturated fat (6%), 84 mg cholesterol, 33 g dietary fiber, 2,149 mg sodium, 1,812 mg calcium

---

FUN TUMMY TRUTH
You produce 1.7 liters of saliva a day and 10,000 gallons in your lifetime.

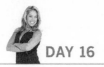

DAY 16

DENISE'S DAILY WISDOM

Anyone who knows me knows that I'm a phone walker. I actually walk pretty quickly while on the phone (sometimes I'm on the treadmill), enough to get slightly (but not noticeably) out of breath. Even just standing—rather than sitting—while talking on the phone has a benefit. The Institute for National Resources in Concord, California, has determined that standing during three 10-minute phone conversations burns 20 calories, whereas sitting during the same conversations burns only 4!

TODAY'S WORKOUT

Core Cardio Blast routine (see pages 168 to 195)

TODAY'S MENU

Breakfast
French Toast (page 273)

Lunch
Just-Like-Chinese-Takeout (page 273)

Snack
Fruit and Cheese Tortilla Wrap: Spread an 8" whole-wheat soft tortilla with 1 wedge spreadable cheese such as Laughing Cow and top with 1 cup sliced strawberries and 2 tablespoons chopped pecans. Roll up to eat.

Dinner
Eat out! At your favorite Mexican restaurant, order the green salad with fajita-style chicken. Ask the server to leave any cheese off the salad and for the dressing on the side. Top your salad with a palm-size amount of chicken and 2 tablespoons of light dressing. Enjoy 12 tortilla chips with salsa from the basket on the table (move the basket away after you portion your chips).

Nutrition Analysis
1,499 calories, 82 g protein (22%), 179 g carbohydrates (49%), 55 g total fat (33%), 11 g saturated fat (7%), 95 mg cholesterol, 43 g dietary fiber, 2,040 mg sodium, 1,047 mg calcium

---

FUN TUMMY TRUTH
Your mouth cools or warms your food, making it a suitable temperature for your stomach.

DAY 17

DENISE'S DAILY WISDOM

I buy organic produce whenever possible. For years, I justified the slightly higher cost of organic food because I knew organic farming practices were more earth-friendly and because I worried that pesticide residues on conventionally grown produce might raise my risk for cancer. Recently, I came across a study that shows organic food may slim your waistline. This animal study showed that the pesticide dieldrin doubles body fat levels in mice. These toxins interfere with fat-burning hormones and thyroid function, which also lowers metabolic rate. These toxins may even lower levels of brain chemicals, making you feel tired and listless.

TODAY'S WORKOUT

A 25-minute power walk

TODAY'S MENU

Breakfast
Applesauce Pancakes (page 274)

Lunch
Artichoke Pizza (page 274)

Snack
1 Pria Bar spread with 2 tablespoons peanut butter

Dinner
1 frozen Amy's Kitchen Vegetable Lasagna (or choose another frozen entrée with 300 calories and less than 6 grams of saturated fat)

6 ounces fat-free Stonyfield Farm Peach, Raspberry, Strawberry, French Vanilla, Black Cherry, or Blueberry yogurt topped with 1 tablespoon chopped walnuts

Nutrition Analysis
1,510 calories, 72 g protein (18%), 200 g carbohydrates (52%), 52 g total fat (32%), 13 g saturated fat (9%), 41 mg cholesterol, 20 g dietary fiber, 2,652 mg sodium, 1,243 mg calcium

---

FUN TUMMY TRUTH
Americans eat more than 2 billion pounds of chocolate a year.

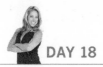

DAY 18

DENISE'S DAILY WISDOM

I'm a mom, so I know how challenging it is to get kids to eat their vegetables. Here's a little secret. Most kids love dips. So serve up a plate of raw veggies (carrots, celery, cauliflower) and some hummus (or any other dip from this plan) and let them dip away! My daughters and their friends love it!

TODAY'S WORKOUT

Core Complete routine (see pages 154 to 167) plus 25 minutes of cardio of your choice

TODAY'S MENU

Breakfast

Southwestern Scrambled Eggs (page 275)

Lunch

Pasta with Corn and Tomato: Combine 1 cup cooked whole wheat pasta, any shape, with ¾ cup cooked corn, 1 tablespoon red wine vinegar, 2 teaspoons extra-virgin olive oil, 1 thinly sliced scallion, and 1 small chopped tomato.

Snack

Waffle with Ricotta Topping: Toast 1 whole grain waffle, fill with ⅓ cup fat-free ricotta cheese mixed with 1 tablespoon maple syrup and 1 teaspoon brown sugar, slice, and eat like a sandwich.

1 cup fat-free milk

Dinner

Teriyaki Swordfish (page 275)

Nutrition Analysis

1,470 calories, 83 g protein (18%), 231 g carbohydrates (52%), 31 g total fat (32%), 5 g saturated fat (9%), 64 mg cholesterol, 31 g dietary fiber, 2,961 mg sodium, 1,033 mg calcium

---

FUN TUMMY TRUTH

In your lifetime, your digestive tract will handle about 50 tons of food.

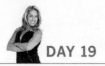

DAY 19

DENISE'S DAILY WISDOM

Worrying does more than put lines on your face; it puts pounds on your middle. When my mind is racing with various to-do lists and worried thoughts, I give myself a 5-minute break—no matter how busy I am—and list all of my worries for the day on a piece of paper. Then I crumple up the paper and toss it—ceremoniously tossing my worries away! Or sometime I just say a little prayer; that always helps.

TODAY'S WORKOUT

Core Cardio Blast routine (see pages 168 to 195)

TODAY'S MENU

Breakfast

1 Tone Your Tummy Type On-the-Go Muffin

1 stick light string cheese

1 apple

1 cup fat-free milk

Lunch

Spinach Dip and Whole Wheat Crackers (page 275)

Snack

4 plain graham cracker squares spread with 2 tablespoons almond butter

Dinner

Falafel (page 276)

Nutrition Analysis

1,541 calories, 68 g protein (18%), 200 g carbohydrates (52%), 58 g total fat (34%), 8 g saturated fat (5%), 34 mg cholesterol, 27 g dietary fiber, 1,863 mg sodium, 1,173 mg calcium

---

FUN TUMMY TRUTH

The human stomach contains neurotransmitters similar to those found in the brain, which is why you sometimes get a "gut" feeling.

The Tummy Type Program

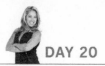

DENISE'S DAILY WISDOM

Did you know that chewing sugarless gum or drinking through a straw can make you appear bloated? These habits tend to fill up the stomach and intestines with air, making your tummy round outward. So if you have an important appearance on a given day where you will be wearing tummy-revealing clothing, put aside the gum and the straw for another day!

TODAY'S WORKOUT

You have the day off from formal exercise, but try to do something fun and active with your family.

TODAY'S MENU

Breakfast
Crunchy Granola Bowl: Combine 6 ounces Stonyfield Farm French Vanilla yogurt with ⅓ cup low-fat granola cereal and 2 tablespoons slivered almonds.

Lunch
Lemon and Dill Chicken with Caesar Salad (page 276)

Snack
4 plain graham crackers dipped in ½ cup fat-free ricotta cheese mixed with 2 tablespoons maple syrup

Dinner
1 Weight Watchers Smart Ones Salisbury Steak (or choose any frozen entrée with 260 calories and less than 6 grams of saturated fat)

1 banana spread with 1 tablespoon peanut butter

Nutrition Analysis
1,479 calories, 82 g protein (22%), 194 g carbohydrates (52%), 46 g total fat (28%), 11 g saturated fat (7%), 140 mg cholesterol, 21 g dietary fiber, 1,969 mg sodium, 1,158 mg calcium

---

FUN TUMMY TRUTH
Just like fingerprints, no two belly buttons are alike.

DENISE'S DAILY WISDOM

Ever notice that when infants breathe, their tummies go up and down? That's because they're breathing deeply and slowly, instead of fast and shallowly (the way many adults breathe). When you breathe shallowly—only with your chest—you don't fully oxygenate your lungs, which makes you feel tired. You also can trigger feelings of stress and anxiety. Deep breathing, on the other hand, tends to make you feel calm and energized. So whenever you find yourself feeling tense—and, as a result, craving something that lies inside your refrigerator—take a moment to breathe deeply. It might just stop a cheat in its tracks!

ASSESS YOUR SUCCESS

Take your measurements or step on the scale. Take another photo of yourself. How much weight have you lost? How many inches have you lost in your waistline?

TAKE TIME TO REFLECT

Wow—3 weeks into the program. I bet you are seeing great results. Take a moment to reflect on how far you've come. By now your clothes are probably fitting better. More important, I bet you are experiencing some of the wonderful benefits of getting in better shape. Do you have more energy? Does exercise feel invigorating? Are you starting to enjoy the tastes of some of the new recipes? Keep it up!

TODAY'S WORKOUT

You have the day off from formal exercise, but try to do something you enjoy that keeps you moving, like gardening.

TODAY'S MENU

Breakfast

Cheddar and Tomato English Muffin: Preheat the oven to 250°F. Top 1 whole grain English muffin with 1 sliced tomato and 2 tablespoons reduced-fat shredded Cheddar cheese.

1 cup fat-free milk

¾ cup grapes

Lunch

Avocado Roll-Up: Fill an 8" whole wheat soft tortilla with ¼ of a sliced cucumber, 2 tablespoons salsa, ½ of a chopped avocado, ¼ cup reduced-fat shredded Cheddar cheese, and 2 tablespoons soft goat cheese. Roll up to eat.

Snack

⅓ cup soy nuts

1 cup strawberries

1 cup fat-free milk

Dinner

Mesquite Chicken Salad (page 276)

Nutrition Analysis

1,471 calories, 87 g protein (24%), 189 g carbohydrates (51%), 47 g total fat (29%), 14 g saturated fat (9%), 72 mg cholesterol, 48 g dietary fiber, 2,629 mg sodium, 1,281 mg calcium

---

FUN TUMMY TRUTH
You burn more calories while sleeping than while watching television.

Week 4 Shopping List

Produce

3 (9-ounce) bags baby spinach leaves

1 regular-size carrot

1 (8-ounce) bag grated carrots*

16 ounces grapes, red or green

1 (4-ounce) sweet potato

1 pear

2 peaches

2 bananas

1 (3-ounce) red potato

3 apples

2 tomatoes, small size such as Roma variety

2 green bell peppers*

1 small orange bell pepper

½ cup mushrooms

2 grapefruit*

1 kiwifruit

1 orange

2 cups raspberries†

½ cup strawberries†

1 cup blackberries†

6 ribs celery†

3 tablespoons lemon juice

2 cups arugula

1 cup romaine lettuce

4 cups spring mix greens

2 cups broccoli†

2 ears of corn, white or yellow

Dairy

1 (6-ounce) container fat-free vanilla yogurt with 140 calories or less and at least 300 milligrams calcium, such as Stonyfield Farm French Vanilla

4 (6-ounce) containers fat-free fruit-flavored yogurt with 140 calories or less and at least 300 milligrams calcium, such as Stonyfield Farm Peach, Raspberry, Strawberry, French Vanilla, Apricot-Mango, Berry Bash, Black Cherry, or Blueberry

1 (6-ounce) container fat-free mocha yogurt with 140 calories or less and at least 300 milligrams calcium, such as Stonyfield Farm Mocha Latte

1 (6-ounce) container fat-free chocolate yogurt with 140 calories or less and at least 300 milligrams calcium, such as Stonyfield Farm Chocolate Underground

1 (6-ounce) fat-free lemon yogurt with no more than 140 calories and at least 300 milligrams calcium, such as Stonyfield Farm Lotsa Lemon

1 (8-ounce) container calcium-fortified orange juice

16 ounces fat-free or 1% fat cottage cheese

½ gallon fat-free milk

Meat/Seafood

1 (4-ounce) piece whitefish such as tilefish or snapper

1 (3-ounce) and 1 (4-ounce) boneless, skinless chicken breasts (7 ounces total)

4 ounces beef tenderloin

*This amount will last through the rest of the 4-week plan.
†Choose either fresh or unsweetened, plain frozen variety.

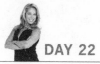

DAY 22

DENISE'S DAILY WISDOM

I know brown rice contains more fiber than white rice and is healthier for my family, but my kids only like white. So I meet them halfway. Whenever we have rice, I mix up a concoction of half brown rice, half white rice. Although this obviously isn't as healthful as 100 percent brown rice, I find it's a compromise that works for the entire family.

TODAY'S WORKOUT

Core Complete routine (see pages 154 to 167) plus 25 minutes of cardio of your choice

TODAY'S MENU

Breakfast
Idaho Potato and Eggs (page 277)

Lunch
Cheese Quesadilla (page 277)

Snack
Fruit Shake (page 278)

Dinner
Beef and Brown Rice (page 278)

Nutrition Analysis
1,533 calories, 106 g protein (27%), 183 g carbohydrates (48%), 44 g total fat (26%), 9 g saturated fat (5%), 113 mg cholesterol, 27 g dietary fiber, 1,671 mg sodium, 1,626 mg calcium

---

FUN TUMMY TRUTH
Your digestive system starts working before you take your first bite of food. The sight and smell of food make glands in your mouth produce saliva.

DAY 23

DENISE'S DAILY WISDOM

Here's a fun way to watch your calorie intake. Keep a portion-control basket on the kitchen counter. Fill it with a lightbulb, a tennis ball, two dice, a ping-pong ball, a ceramic egg, a hockey puck, and an old computer mouse. Now you have visual cues for portion sizes for everything from a baked potato (computer mouse) and bagel (hockey puck) to cheese (two dice), cooked veggies (lightbulb), and fruit (tennis ball).

TODAY'S WORKOUT

Core Cardio Blast routine (see pages 168 to 195)

TODAY'S MENU

Breakfast
Nutty Oatmeal: Make oatmeal with ½ cup dry oatmeal and ½ cup fat-free milk, and mix in 1 tablespoon peanut butter and 1 tablespoon peanuts.

Lunch
Orzo Carrot Pecan Salad (page 278)

Snack
Berry Chocolate Yogurt: Top 6 ounces fat-free Stonyfield Farm Chocolate Underground yogurt with ½ cup raspberries and 2 tablespoons chopped pecans.

1 cup fat-free milk

Dinner
White Bean and Tuna Salad (page 279)

Nutrition Analysis
1,536 calories, 76 g protein (19%), 206 g carbohydrates (54%), 49 g total fat (28%), 11 g saturated fat (6%), 79 mg cholesterol, 25 g dietary fiber, 1,159 mg sodium, 1,139 mg calcium

---

FUN TUMMY TRUTH
It takes roughly 6 hours for your stomach to break down a high-fat meal and about 2 hours to break down a high-carbohydrate meal.

The Tummy Type Program

DAY 24

DENISE'S DAILY WISDOM

I've never liked artificial sweeteners. I'm one of those people who wants the foods I eat to come from nature and not from a chemistry lab. However, I didn't have any real proof about the dangers of artificial sweeteners—until now. Emerging research shows that foods and beverages that contain artificial sweeteners can throw off your own natural ability to monitor calories, increasing your risk of overeating.

TODAY'S WORKOUT

A 25-minute power walk

TODAY'S MENU

Breakfast
Quick Peach Cobbler (page 279)

Lunch
Waldorf Salad (page 279)

Snack
Protein-Packed Smoothie: In a blender, combine 1 tablespoon wheat germ, 1 cup fat-free milk, 3 ounces tofu with calcium sulfate, 1 cup blackberries (for a really thick, frosty smoothie, don't thaw berries if using frozen), and ½ teaspoon almond or vanilla extract.

Dinner
Sesame Chicken (page 280)

Nutrition Analysis
1,451 calories, 73 g protein (20%), 191 g carbohydrates (52%), 50 g total fat (31%), 6 g saturated fat (4%), 71mg cholesterol, 30 g dietary fiber, 521 mg sodium, 1,197 mg calcium

---

FUN TUMMY TRUTH
During your lifetime, you will eat the weight of six full-grown elephants.

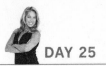

DENISE'S DAILY WISDOM

I love yogurt. In addition to a wealth of tummy-slimming calcium, most varieties also deliver plenty of live and active bacteria cultures for healthy digestion (which prevents bloating). Most commercial yogurts, however, contain a lot of added sugar. Yogurts that advertise "fruit on the bottom" or "fruit flavoring contain very little—if any—real fruit. To reduce my intake of added sugars (and calories), I usually buy plain, unflavored yogurt and mix in my own favorite berries and fruit.

TODAY'S WORKOUT

Core Complete routine (see pages 154 to 167) plus 25 minutes of cardio of your choice

TODAY'S MENU

Breakfast

Chunky Peanut Wrap: Open an 8" whole wheat soft tortilla, lay 1 peeled banana in the tortilla, sprinkle with 1 tablespoon peanuts, and roll up to eat.

1 cup fat-free milk

Lunch

Salmon Caesar Salad (page 280)

Snack

1 Kellogg's All-Bran Cereal Bar (any flavor)

¾ cup grapes

6 ounces fat-free plain Stonyfield Farm yogurt

Dinner

Pasta with Goat Cheese (page 280)

Nutrition Analysis

1,513 calories, 72 g protein (19%), 181 g carbohydrates (48%), 55 g total fat (33%), 15 g saturated fat (9%), 97 mg cholesterol, 43 g dietary fiber, 1,324 mg sodium, 994 mg calcium

---

FUN TUMMY TRUTH

Your abdominal muscles support your spine. The stronger your abdomen, the less your back muscles must work to hold you upright—and the less back discomfort you will feel.

DENISE'S DAILY WISDOM

Always keep an abundance of frozen fruit and vegetables in your freezer. Frozen at the peak of freshness, frozen produce allows you to quickly round out any meal. For instance, toss frozen veggies into soups and stews, microwave for a side dish, or thaw and dip into low-fat salad dressing for snacks. The frozen fruits are ideal for smoothies, desserts, or mixed into yogurt.

TODAY'S WORKOUT

Core Cardio Blast routine (see pages 168 to 195)

TODAY'S MENU

Breakfast

Almond Toast and Apple: Toast 1 slice of rye bread and spread with 1 tablespoon almond butter, and slice an apple and spread with 1 tablespoon almond butter.

Lunch

1 Amy's Kitchen Indian Vegetable Korma (or any frozen entrée with 300 calories and less than 5 grams of saturated fat)

½ cup grapes

1 stick light string cheese

Snack

Mocha Fruit Bowl: Combine 6 ounces low-fat Stonyfield Farm Mocha Latte yogurt with ½ cup raspberries, ½ cup strawberries, and 20 chocolate-covered espresso beans.

1 cup fat-free milk

Dinner

Spinach and Feta Pizza (page 281)

Nutrition Analysis

1,446 calories, 61 g protein (18%), 204 g carbohydrates (55%), 49 g total fat (29%), 10 g saturated fat (6%), 48 mg cholesterol, 23 g dietary fiber, 2,313 mg sodium, 1,281 mg calcium

---

FUN TUMMY TRUTH

You can't physically taste your food until your saliva dissolves it.

DAY 27

DENISE'S DAILY WISDOM

The Tone Your Tummy Type program recommends that you power walk on a regular basis. If you're in a hurry, turn your power walk into a multitasking adventure. Instead of driving to the dry cleaner, then the bank, then the post office, then the drugstore, find a section of town where businesses are grouped fairly close and do your walking as you run your errands, returning often to your car to drop things off.

TODAY'S WORKOUT

You have the day off from your regular plan exercise, but try to do something fun, like bike riding or hiking with your family.

TODAY'S MENU

Breakfast

1 Tone Your Tummy Type On-the-Go Muffin

6 ounces fat-free Stonyfield Farm Peach, Raspberry, Strawberry, French Vanilla, Apricot-Mango, Berry Bash, Black Cherry, or Blueberry yogurt mixed with 1 chopped pear

Lunch

Big Chef Salad (page 281)

Snack

Baby Vegetables and Parmesan Dip: In a blender, combine 1 cup 1% or fat-free cottage cheese, ¼ cup salsa, and 2 tablespoons Parmesan cheese. Dip with 10 baby carrots and 1 sliced baby zucchini.

Dinner

Apricot Fish with Baked Sweet Potato Fries (page 281)

Nutrition Analysis

1,556 calories, 103 g protein (26%), 187 g carbohydrates (48%), 49 g total fat (28%), 14 g saturated fat (8%), 148 mg cholesterol, 27 g dietary fiber, 3,387 mg sodium, 1,306 mg calcium

---

FUN TUMMY TRUTH

The average person has 9,000 tastebuds that line the surface of the tongue, throat, and roof of the mouth.

DENISE'S DAILY WISDOM

If the only way you can find out what happens next in a book is to slip on the earphones and head out for your walk, I guarantee you'll walk more often. These days, you can download books online, borrow books on tape or CD from the local library, or buy them in bookstores. Consider it exercising your mind as well as your body.

ASSESS YOUR SUCCESS

Take your measurements or step on the scale. Take another photo of yourself. How much weight have you lost? How many inches have you lost in your waistline?

TAKE TIME TO REFLECT

You did it! I hope you feel better, have more energy, and got great results. My goal for you is to get "hooked" on eating right and exercising. Healthy habits are the keys.

TODAY'S WORKOUT

It's your "free day." Stretch to help relax and refresh you for the coming week.

TODAY'S MENU

Breakfast
¾ cup muesli (such as Healthy Choice Mueslix Raisin and Almond Crunch with Dates or Kellogg's Mueslix) topped with ½ cup cubed pineapple and ½ cup fat-free milk

½ cup fat-free milk

Lunch
Tuna with Parmesan Spinach (page 282)

Snack
1 apple spread with 1 tablespoon peanut butter

6 ounces fat-free Stonyfield Farm Peach, Raspberry, Strawberry, French Vanilla, Apricot-Mango, Berry Bash, Black Cherry, or Blueberry yogurt

Dinner
Grilled Chicken with Arugula Salad and Maple Corn (page 282)

Nutrition Analysis
1,499 calories, 99 g protein (26%), 195 g carbohydrates (52%), 42 g total fat (25%), 8 g saturated fat (5%), 126 mg cholesterol, 39 g dietary fiber, 1,903 mg sodium, 1,161 mg calcium

---

FUN TUMMY TRUTH

If you stretched your intestines end to end, they would cover 26 feet.

PHASE 2 SUCCESS

Congratulations! You've come to the unofficial end of phase 2. I call it the unofficial end because phase 2 really lasts the rest of your life! Turn to Chapter 14 to find out everything you need to know to stick with the Tone Your Tummy Type program; enhance and maintain your results; and make it a fun, tasty, and healthy part of the rest of your life.

14 A LIFETIME OF FIRM, SEXY ABS

**Everything You Need to Know
to Keep Your Tummy Flat and Firm Forever**

You've almost reached the end of the Tone Your Tummy Type program. You've worked hard! You've put in the required exercise. You've tried new recipes, shopped for new ingredients, and shifted to a new way of eating. You've even made a few lifestyle changes. And, more important, you've seen the results of that effort. You have shrunk inches off your waistline, seen pounds erased off the scale, and dropped a dress size or two—or three. You've flattened your tummy—finally—and now feel confident wearing just about anything. No more long, bulky shirts. No more elastic waistbands.

More important, you feel great. That nagging back pain has subsided. Your stronger abdomen now gives you the core strength you need to lift, pull, reach, and bend. You're a true superwoman. Finally, by shrinking that dangerous tummy fat, you've literally grown younger, adding many extra years to your life span!

Now you want to stay this way! With 28 or more days of Tone Your Tummy Type eating and exercising under your belt, you may be wondering, "Where do I go from here?" And that's what you'll find in the following pages.

To answer that question, you first must decide whether you want to keep losing weight or whether you have reached your goal. If you still would like to lose a bit more tummy fat, you will continue to follow the Keep-On-Losing Phase. Just because the meal plan only spans 2 weeks doesn't mean phase 2 ends on Day 28! To continue to lose tummy fat, choose one of the following options.

Option 1: Go back to Day 15 in your planner in Chapter 13, and continue to repeat the 2 weeks of meals and exercise prescriptions until you reach your weight-loss goal.

Option 2: Mix and match your favorite meals and snacks from phase 2 (you may even use ones from phase 1 if you'd like). Continue to follow the phase 2 exercise routines.

Either of those methods will help you to continue to lose tummy fat until you reach your goal. In the pages that follow, you'll find out how to maintain your success after you've reached your goal.

TONE YOUR TUMMY FOR LIFE

To sustain your firm, flat tummy, you will need to preserve certain elements of the Tone Your Tummy Type program for good. You need not do as many tummy-toning exercises as you have up until this point, but you deserve the lasting success that will come with continued effort and attention to your diet.

To fend off fat gain and keep that tummy firm, do the following:

Do 3 to 5 minutes of tummy-firming moves a day. Even as I near my 50th birthday, this is the maximum amount of time I spend on my abs to keep them in shape. The longer 10-minute Core Complete routine you did for phases 1 and 2 helped to strengthen your entire midsection. Now that you've completely firmed those muscles to the max, you can step back your efforts. I recommend you do your tummy-firming moves first thing in the morning—right after getting out of bed. It will help you to start your day on the right foot. Each morning, pick from the moves shown in the phase 1 and phase 2 Core Complete routines, making sure to choose moves that work each part of your midsection: the front of your tummy, your waistline, your back, and your transverse abdominis deep in your tummy. Here are a few short sample routines that I do to maintain a flat tummy.

* Lower-tummy firmer (page 115), heel tap (page 156), Pilates T-stand (beginner or full version, pages 120 and 159)

* Crunch on ball (page 122), back strengthener I (page 119), obliques firmer (page 79), lower-tummy firmer (page 115)

* Straight-leg crunch I or II (pages 116 and 158), Pilates single-leg stretch (page 117), roll-out I or II (pages 123 and 165), standing Pilates swimming (page 141)

* Pilates beginner roll-up (page 114), swan (page 149), plank I (page 148), Pilates crisscross I (page 146)

* Lower-tummy and pelvic-floor strengthener on the ball (page 157), back strengthener II (page 160), low hover II (page 118)

* Pilates double-leg stretch (page 162), waistline slimmer (page 161), back strengthener II (page 160)

* Waistline chop on the ball (page 163), tummy tuck (page 164), crunch on ball (page 122)

Continue to follow tips described for your personal tummy type. Periodically retake the tummy type quiz in Chapter 3. Over time, your age, health, or lifestyle may place you in a different type category than what you were in when you initially tackled the program. For example, you may initially have used this program to firm up your abdomen after a pregnancy. Later in life, after menopause, you may need the tips for the Peri/Postmenopause Tummy Type instead. Every so often, review the chapter that describes your tummy type. Make sure to *always* follow the Top Tummy Type Tactic. The other useful tactics are optional, but if you notice your results slipping, consider incorporating more of these tactics into your lifestyle.

Eat according to Tone Your Tummy Type principles. You may continue to use the precise recipes and meal suggestions for phase 2 of the plan as long as you'd like. If you'd like to branch out and create your own personal Tone Your Tummy Type recipes, follow this basic formula.

* Make sure that 98 percent of what you eat comes from real foods found in nature. Try to limit your intake of processed and refined foods, added sugars, and trans fats (see third bullet) as much as possible.

* Make fruits and vegetables the cornerstones of every meal. They should account for half of every plate of food you eat.

* Focus on healthful fats found in olive oil, nuts, fish, avocado, and olives. Try to eliminate trans fats (found in processed foods). Scale back on saturated fats (found in animal products) as much as possible, but not so much that your food becomes unpalatable. For example, you might switch from cheese made from whole milk to low-fat cheese, but not to fat-free cheese, which tastes rubbery and does not melt easily. On the other hand, you might easily switch to fat-free milk or yogurt. For meat, look to skinless chicken breast, fish, egg whites, and very lean beef (such as sirloin). Use the recipes from phases 1 and 2 for lean protein ideas.

* Keep an eye on your portions. Use the suggested meals and snacks in phase 2 as a rough guide for portion sizes. The suggested meals and snacks in this phase will help you to see what reasonable portions look like.

Continue to add lifestyle movement to each day. Never take the elevator or escalator. Walk your errands rather than driving whenever possible. Walk while talking on the phone, and generally try to stay in motion as much as physically possible.

Follow the cardio and toning recommendations for your type. Some tummy types need more formal exercise than others. For example, if you are postmenopausal, make it your goal to strength-train or do some form of cardio for 45 minutes 5 days a week. You may continue to use the Core Cardio Blast routine outlined in this book, or you may branch out, getting inspiration from fitness DVDs, fitness television shows, or fitness classes.

SECRETS OF LASTING SUCCESS

Believe in yourself. You will maintain your results. You see, I'm a big believer in positive thinking. The more confident you feel about your future success, the more likely you'll be successful in the future.

To help increase your chances of lasting success, I'd like to tell you about some exciting research. Scientists for years have been trying to understand why some people manage to lose weight and keep it off—whereas so many others do not. So, a number of scientists at a number of different institutions around the world have been conducting studies to discover the solution to that perplexing issue. Below is what they have found.

Consider taking a yoga class. In a study of overweight people in their fifties, participants who took yoga lost weight over a 10-year period. Participants who did not practice yoga gained an average of 13 pounds over the same time period. The researchers cautioned that yoga exerts no magical effects on the metabolism, nor does it burn high amounts of calories. It may aid weight maintenance, however, by helping you to stay more in tune with your body, your eating habits, and your negative habits. In particular, the internal focus that yoga promotes may help you to become more in tune with your body's natural cues of when to eat and when to stop eating.

Sit down to eat. A German study of 7,000 people who lost weight and maintained that weight loss for at least a year determined that sitting down to eat helps to prevent the mindless munching that tends to lead to weight gain.

Shop with a list. The same German study mentioned above found that shopping lists help you avoid buying fattening foods.

Exercise religiously. The longer you exercise, the more confident you will feel about your ability to exercise and, consequently, the more you will enjoy exercising. As a side benefit, research shows that this exercise-induced confidence spills over into your eating habits. Researchers have determined that the more confident you feel about your exercise habits, the more in control you will feel about your eating. You will feel more determined to eat only the foods you plan to eat and when you plan to eat them.

Never skip breakfast. It really is the most important meal of your day. Almost 80 percent of the registrants in the National Weight Control Registry—which studies the habits of adults who have lost 30 pounds or more and kept it off for 1 year or longer—eat breakfast every day.

Buy a scale. The National Weight Control Registry finds the majority of people who successfully lose weight and keep it off for more than a year weigh themselves at least once a week, and 38 percent hit the scales daily. The reason? Weighing yourself provides important information about where you are, where you need to go, and whether recent activities are benefiting or harming your efforts.

Stick to single-serving packages. If you buy tiny containers of ice cream, mini packs of cookies, small yogurts, and individually wrapped cheeses, you're much less likely to go overboard.

Keep a food journal. Many of the participants in the National Weight Control Registry use food journals to stay on track. Writing down what you eat will keep you honest. It also might make you think twice before eating that jelly doughnut!

ENJOY YOUR TONED TUMMY!

I'm so proud of you for making the commitment to shrinking tummy fat. You've seen your efforts pay off in real, tangible results. You can zip up your jeans, feel confident tucking in your shirts, and may even be known to bare your tummy from time to time.

More important than the physical benefits, however, are the benefits to your health. The exercises and eating strategies that you followed to shrink tummy fat and firm tummy flab have provided you with a healthier body, one that is more capable of resisting disease. You've reduced your risk for developing heart disease, diabetes, and cancer. You've improved your health and fitness. You have more energy, feel happier, and can enjoy life to the fullest.

You've found the answer. Enjoy your new tummy and all the health and happiness possible! Congratulations and keep it up!

15 THE CORE DIET RECIPES

Delicious, Quick-and-Easy Recipes;
Convenient Frozen Dinners; and Restaurant Meals
Specially Designed to Slim Your Midsection

I love healthful, wholesome foods, but, like you, I'm very busy and don't have a lot of time for gourmet cooking. I'm also the mom of two girls—one a tween and the other a teen—who serve as my personal sounding boards regarding the taste and palatability of each meal and snack I dish up. For these reasons, I'm constantly looking for quick-and-easy, family-friendly healthful foods.

I'm excited to tell you that plenty of snacks and meals meet these strict requirements. When you're a busy, on-the-go mom, you do not have to settle for typical options like hot dogs, snack crackers, and fast food. You and your family can do better!

Even the most hapless cook or time-starved career woman can prepare the tasty and easy-to-throw-together recipes that appear in the following pages. These snack ideas and recipes are based on the very meals and snacks that I cook up for my family every day. To ensure that my personal family favorites were as healthful as possible, I worked with Chevy Chase, Maryland–

based nutritionist Tracy Olgeaty Gensler, MS, RD. She analyzed all the recipes for nutrient content, helping me to make sure each recipe contains a wealth of tummy-slimming ingredients, tastes delicious, and is simple and easy to prepare. Her tips and suggestions helped to elevate the Austin family favorites to a whole new level of simplicity and wholesomeness.

I'm very conscious about taste, and I believe in flexibility. For example, many nutritionists recommend using a trans-free tub margarine instead of butter or regular margarine. Although I know these trans-free margarines are probably healthier than butter, I've resisted using them. What can I say? I love the taste of butter, and neither regular margarine nor trans-free margarine comes close to replicating that taste. At the same time, I know butter is high in saturated fat, which you need to minimize in order to trim tummy fat. Tracy suggested a light butter with canola oil by Land O'Lakes. I tried it and am happy to report that it tastes great! A 1-tablespoon serving has just 2 grams of saturated fat, compared with 7 grams for regular butter. You'll find this butter in many of my recipes.

THE JUMP-START CORE DIET RECIPES

For your convenience, I've listed the phase 1 recipes in the order that you will be using them. In the following list, you'll find some vegetarian options, as well as a variety of recipes for pasta, pizza, beef, soup, and salads. For breakfast, you'll find skillet options as well as cereal, waffles, and yogurt. Mmm, yummy!

Tone Your Tummy Type On-the-Go Muffins

Prep: 8 minutes *Cook: 30 minutes* *Makes 15 muffins*

1½	cups oatmeal
1	cup whole wheat pastry flour
⅓	cup sunflower seeds
¼	cup flax meal
½	teaspoon caraway seeds
2	teaspoons baking powder
½	teaspoon salt
⅓	cup light brown sugar
1	omega-3 egg
⅓	cup sunflower oil
1	cup fat-free milk mixed with 2 teaspoons lemon juice to make "buttermilk"

Preheat the oven to 350°F. Line muffin cups with muffin wrappers. In a bowl, combine the oatmeal, flour, sunflower seeds, flax meal, caraway seeds, baking powder, salt, and sugar. In another bowl, whisk together the egg, oil, and "buttermilk" and add to the dry ingredients, stirring until just blended. Some lumps will remain. Spoon into the muffin cups, filling each cup ¾ full, and bake for about 30 minutes. Remove muffins to a cooling rack and freeze in a zipper-lock bag for up to 2 months. When ready to serve, defrost a muffin on the counter for about 15 minutes, or use the defrost feature of your microwave and defrost for about 30 seconds.

Variation: Add 2 tablespoons of mini chocolate chips for only an extra 10 calories per muffin.

Asian Chicken with Couscous

Prep: 36 minutes   *Cook: 18 minutes*   *Servings: 1*

In a zipper-lock bag, combine 1 tablespoon reduced-sodium soy sauce and 2 tablespoons calcium-fortified orange juice with ½ teaspoon each minced garlic and ground ginger. Add a 4-ounce raw chicken breast to the bag and marinate in the refrigerator for 30 minutes to overnight. Lightly coat a skillet with olive oil cooking spray and heat over low to medium heat. Add the chicken and cook on both sides until cooked through, about 7 to 9 minutes. Serve with 1 cup cooked whole wheat couscous mixed with 1 diced tomato, ¼ teaspoon black pepper, and 1 teaspoon extra-virgin olive oil.

Orange-Glazed Salmon with Pecans

Prep: 5 minutes   *Cook: 17 minutes*   *Servings: 1*

Preheat oven to 400°F. Lightly coat a baking dish with olive oil cooking spray and add a 4-ounce piece of salmon. Drizzle the salmon with 1 tablespoon white wine and 1 teaspoon reduced-sodium soy sauce and bake for 8 to 10 minutes. In the meantime, cook 1 cup broccoli florets and set aside. Lightly coat a small saucepan with olive oil cooking spray and heat over medium-high heat with ¼ cup calcium-fortified orange juice, 1 teaspoon orange peel, and 1 teaspoon cooking sherry. Stir frequently for 3 to 5 minutes, until the sauce thickens. Drizzle over the cooked broccoli and the salmon, then top the salmon with 1 tablespoon chopped pecans and the broccoli with 2 tablespoons shredded reduced-fat mozzarella cheese. Serve with 1 sliced kiwifruit.

Pinto Bean Bowl

Prep: 4 minutes   *Servings: 1*

Combine 1 cup canned pinto beans (rinsed and drained) with ¼ cup chopped white or yellow onion, ½ teaspoon minced garlic, 2 teaspoons extra-virgin olive oil, 1 teaspoon lemon juice, and 1 tablespoon balsamic vinegar.

Parmesan Turkey Pasta with Vegetables

Prep: 9 minutes   *Cook: 25 minutes*   *Servings: 1*

Heat 1 teaspoon extra-virgin olive oil in a saucepan over low to medium heat. Add 3 ounces ground turkey breast and heat until cooked through, about 6 to 7 minutes. Remove the cooked turkey to a bowl. In the same saucepan as you cooked the turkey, add 1 cup broccoli florets, ¾ cup prepared cream of celery soup such as Campbell's Healthy Request Cream of Celery Soup or 60 calories of another brand, ½ cup sliced mushrooms, ½ cup fat-free milk, 1 minced garlic clove, ¼ teaspoon each onion powder and ground black pepper, and 1 tablespoon Parmesan cheese. Turn up the heat and bring the mixture to a boil, then reduce the heat to low, cover, and simmer for 8 minutes. Add ½ cup cooked whole wheat pasta and cooked turkey breast to the saucepan to warm before serving. Serve with 6 ounces fat-free Greek yogurt topped with 1 tablespoon raisins.

Cherry Smoothie

Prep: 3 minutes   *Servings: 1*

In a blender, combine 1 cup fresh or unsweetened, frozen cherries with 6 ounces fat-free plain Stonyfield Farm yogurt. Top with ½ cup Kashi Good Friends cereal (or 60 calories of your favorite high-fiber cereal) and 1 tablespoon slivered almonds.

Poppy Chicken Salad

Prep: 4 minutes   *Cook: 10 minutes*   *Servings: 1*

Combine 2 ounces sliced deli chicken breast cut into small pieces, 1 diced tomato, 1 table-spoon light canola oil mayonnaise, 1 teaspoon honey, 1 tablespoon balsamic vinegar, and ½ teaspoon poppy seeds. Prepare 1 hard-cooked egg, slice in half as you would a deviled egg, remove the yolk (feed to your pet if you'd like), and fill each half with 1 tablespoon hummus. Place the chicken salad and hummus deviled egg on top of 2 cups romaine let-tuce and serve with a side of 6 ounces fat-free Stonyfield Farm Peach, Raspberry, Straw-berry, or Apricot-Mango yogurt.

Pasta with Chickpeas

Prep: 4 minutes   *Cook: 10 minutes*   *Servings: 1*

Prepare ½ cup cooked whole wheat pasta, any shape. Toss the cooked pasta with 1 table-spoon extra-virgin olive oil, 1 tablespoon Parmesan cheese, ½ teaspoon dried basil, 1 tea-spoon minced garlic, 1 diced tomato, and ⅔ cup canned chickpeas (rinsed and drained).

Maple Ricotta Cereal Bowl

Prep: 2 minutes   *Servings: 1*

Combine ½ cup fat-free ricotta cheese with 1 tablespoon maple syrup, 1 teaspoon honey, and ½ teaspoon ground cinnamon. Mix well and add ¼ cup Kashi Good Friends cereal (or ¼ cup Cheerios or 30 calories of your favorite high-fiber cereal) and 1 tablespoon chopped walnuts.

Pita Triangles and Bean Dip

Prep: 2 minutes   *Servings: 1*

Combine ⅔ cup fat-free refried beans with ¼ cup fat-free sour cream, 2 teaspoons extra-virgin olive oil, and ¼ teaspoon each chili powder and ground cumin. Use as a dip for 1 toasted 6" whole wheat pita, cut into triangles. Serve with 1 apple.

Mild Cajun Fish Stew

Prep: 6 minutes   *Cook: 38 minutes*   *Servings: 1*

Prepare ½ cup cooked brown rice and set aside. Coat a skillet with cooking spray and heat over low to medium heat. Add ¼ cup chopped onion, 1 minced garlic clove, 1 chopped green bell pepper, 1 can (8 ounces) no-salt-added chopped tomatoes (include liquid), 1 teaspoon canola oil, and ⅛ teaspoon each dried basil, thyme flakes, ground black pepper, and paprika. Add 1 shake of cayenne pepper. Cover skillet and simmer the mixture for 20 minutes over medium heat, then turn up the heat to bring to a boil. Add 6 ounces chopped halibut, sole, or flounder fillet and cook for 4 to 5 minutes. Serve immediately over the brown rice.

Apple, Potato, and Egg Skillet

Prep: 5 minutes   *Cook: 17 minutes*   *Servings: 1*

Lightly coat a skillet with olive oil cooking spray. Heat over low to medium heat. Add ¼ cup chopped white or yellow onion, 1 chopped apple (with skin), and a 2-ounce potato with skin, grated. Cook for 10 minutes, stirring frequently, until the potatoes turn golden brown. Add 2 tablespoons each shredded reduced-fat Cheddar cheese and fat-free sour cream, and 2 lightly beaten egg whites. Pour off excess water as the egg and potato cook. Cover the skillet and continue to cook for 4 to 6 minutes, until the eggs are set. Serve with 1 cup fat-free milk.

Honey and Garlic Chicken with Brown Rice

Prep: 37 minutes   *Cook: 16 minutes*   *Servings: 1*

In a zipper-lock bag, combine 1 tablespoon each honey and lemon juice, 1 minced garlic clove (about 1 teaspoon), and 1 teaspoon reduced-sodium soy sauce. Add 2 ounces raw chicken breast to the bag and marinate in the refrigerator for 30 minutes to overnight. Lightly coat a skillet with olive oil cooking spray and heat over low to medium heat. Add the chicken and cook on both sides until cooked through, about 5 to 6 minutes. Serve with ½ cup cooked brown rice topped with 2 teaspoons toasted pine nuts, and 1 chopped nectarine mixed into 6 ounces fat-free plain Stonyfield Farm yogurt.

Cucumber with Creamy Tahini Spread

Prep: 5 minutes   *Servings: 1*

In a blender, combine ¼ cup 1% or fat-free cottage cheese with 1 tablespoon tahini butter and ⅛ teaspoon dried parsley. Slice 1 small cucumber and dip the slices in the spread. Serve with 1 cup fat-free milk.

Hummus and Baked Chips

Prep: 7 minutes   *Servings: 1*

Combine ½ cup chickpeas, ⅓ cup hummus, 1 diced tomato, and ⅛ teaspoon black pepper. Dip with 9 baked tortilla chips, about ½ ounce chips. Serve with 1 sliced kiwifruit.

Bell Pepper and Carrots with Onion Dip

Prep: 3 minutes   *Cook: 4 minutes*   *Dip servings: 2*

Lightly coat a saucepan with olive oil cooking spray and heat over low to medium heat. Add 1 cup chopped white or yellow onion. Sauté the onion for 3 to 4 minutes, or until translucent. Combine the onion with 1 cup fat-free sour cream, ¼ teaspoon each onion powder and black pepper, and 2 teaspoons light canola oil mayonnaise. Divide dip in half. Serve half with 10 baby carrots and 1 sliced green bell pepper. Store the other half of the dip in the refrigerator; it will keep fresh for up to 3 days.

Beef Tenderloin and Mediterranean Spinach

Prep: 8 minutes   *Cook: 29 minutes*   *Servings: 1*

Preheat the oven to 350°F. Lightly coat a baking dish with olive oil cooking spray. Add a 4-ounce beef tenderloin steak. Tenderize by piercing the steak 6 to 8 times. Cover the beef with 1 tablespoon balsamic vinegar and ½ teaspoon each ground oregano and ground black pepper. Bake for 25 minutes. Lightly coat a skillet with olive oil cooking spray, add 1 teaspoon extra-virgin olive oil, and heat over low to medium heat. Add ¼ cup chopped onion and sauté for 1 to 2 minutes, then add 2 cups baby spinach leaves, 1 tablespoon balsamic vinegar, and 1 minced garlic clove. Sauté for 2 minutes, or until the spinach begins to wilt. Remove from the heat and top with ¼ cup reduced-fat feta cheese. Serve with the beef tenderloin. Serve with 1 cup fat-free milk.

DAY 7
Chicken Pita

Prep: 3 minutes   *Servings: 1*

Open an 8" whole wheat pita and spread with 1 teaspoon Dijon mustard. Add 3 ounces sliced cooked chicken breast and a sprinkle of black pepper. Top with ⅓ cup salsa and 3 tablespoons shredded reduced-fat Cheddar cheese.

DAY 8
Tortilla with Sunflower Cucumber Spread

Prep: 3 minutes   *Servings: 1*

Combine 3 ounces fat-free plain Stonyfield Farm yogurt, ⅛ of a chopped cucumber, and 1 tablespoon sunflower seeds. Spread between two 8" whole wheat tortillas. Fill with ⅛ sliced cucumber and 1 tablespoon soft goat cheese.

DAY 8
London Broil Chicken with Pesto

Prep: 35 minutes   *Cook: 19 minutes*   *Servings: 1*

In a zipper-lock bag, combine 1 tablespoon each lemon juice, red cooking wine, and Worcestershire sauce. Add a 3-ounce raw chicken breast to the bag and marinate in the refrigerator for 30 minutes to overnight. Lightly coat a skillet with olive oil cooking spray and heat over low to medium heat. Add the chicken and cook on both sides for 7 to 9 minutes or until cooked through. Place 1 tablespoon toasted slivered almonds, 1 teaspoon extra-virgin olive oil, 1 garlic clove, 1 tablespoon fresh basil leaves, and a sprinkle each of black pepper and nutmeg in a food processor and blend all ingredients into a coarse paste, creating a pesto. Spoon the pesto over ½ cup cooked whole wheat pasta. Serve with 6 ounces fat-free plain Stonyfield Farm yogurt.

Crunchy Salmon Cakes

Prep: 7 minutes   *Cook: 23 minutes*   *Servings: 1*

Preheat the oven to 350°F. Lightly coat a baking dish with plain cooking spray. In a small bowl, combine 4 ounces raw salmon with 3 tablespoons seasoned bread crumbs, 1 tablespoon light canola oil mayonnaise, 1 tablespoon lemon juice, 1 egg white, 1 sliced spring onion, and ¼ teaspoon Dijon mustard. Form into 2 patties, place in the baking dish, and bake for 20 minutes. Serve with 1 small ear corn or ¾ cup cooked corn.

Salmon and Veggies with Spicy Ranch Sauce

Prep: 10 minutes   *Cook: 21 minutes*   *Servings: 1*

Preheat the oven to 350°F. Lightly coat a baking dish with plain cooking spray. Place a 3-ounce piece of raw salmon in the middle, and surround the salmon with 1 diced tomato and 1 small sliced zucchini. Sprinkle with ⅛ teaspoon black pepper and bake for 15 minutes. Remove from the oven. Spread the fish with 1 teaspoon Dijon mustard, drizzle 2 tablespoons light ranch dressing over the vegetables and fish, and return to the oven for 3 to 4 minutes. Serve with 1 toasted whole wheat pita spread with 1 tablespoon light canola oil butter.

Grilled Mushrooms, Tomato, and Mozzarella on Pumpernickel

Prep: 5 minutes   *Cook: 7 minutes*   *Servings: 1*

Lightly coat a skillet with olive oil cooking spray and heat over low to medium heat. Add ½ cup sliced mushrooms, ½ cup sliced tomato, and ¼ teaspoon onion powder and sauté for 3 to 4 minutes, stirring frequently. Then add 3 tablespoons reduced-fat mozzarella cheese and heat for 1 minute. Top 1 slice of pumpernickel toast with the mixture. Serve with 1 cup fat-free milk.

Cabbage-Apple Salad

Prep: 11 minutes   *Servings: 1*

In a medium bowl, combine 2 cups shredded prepared coleslaw greens with 1 tablespoon light canola oil mayonnaise, 1 teaspoon honey, 1 tablespoon balsamic vinegar, 4 ounces fat-free plain Stonyfield Farm yogurt, and ½ teaspoon poppy seeds. Add 1 chopped apple and 3 tablespoons chopped walnuts.

Ratatouille

Prep: 11 minutes   *Cook: 22 minutes*   *Servings: 1*

Preheat the oven to 350°F. Lightly coat a baking dish with olive oil cooking spray. Add ½ cup sliced green pepper, ½ cup zucchini slices, 2 tablespoons chopped white or yellow onion, ¼ cup sliced mushrooms, and 1 diced tomato. Top with ⅓ cup pasta sauce, ¼ cup shredded reduced-fat mozzarella cheese, and ¼ teaspoon dried oregano. Bake for 20 minutes. Serve with 1 whole wheat pita toasted and topped with 1 tablespoon light canola oil butter, and 1 cup fat-free milk.

Philadelphia Beef

Prep: 6 minutes   *Cook: 4 minutes*   *Servings: 1*

Preheat the oven to 200°F. Open 1 whole wheat roll and place on a cookie sheet. Spread the roll with 1 tablespoon light canola oil mayonnaise and top with 3 ounces lean deli roast beef such as Healthy Choice brand, 1 slice soy cheese, ½ cup sliced white or yellow onion, and ¼ cup sliced mushrooms. Bake for 3 to 4 minutes, or until the cheese melts.

Orange Roughy and Arugula Blackberry Salad

Prep: 9 minutes   *Cook: 27 minutes*   *Servings: 1*

Preheat the oven to 400°F. Lightly coat a baking sheet with plain cooking spray. In a zipper-lock bag, add 1 ounce dry cornbread mix and ⅛ teaspoon each cayenne pepper and black pepper. Add a 4-ounce orange roughy fillet to the bag, shake to coat well, and place the fish on the baking sheet. Bake for 20 to 25 minutes. Make a salad with 2 cups arugula; ½ cup fresh or frozen, unsweetened blackberries; and 2 tablespoons light dressing such as raspberry vinaigrette (about 80 calories' worth). Top the salad with homemade croutons. To make the croutons, toast 1 slice pumpernickel bread spread with 1 tablespoon light canola oil butter and sprinkled with ¼ teaspoon dried basil, then cut into squares.

Chili Soup

Prep: 7 minutes   *Cook: 24 minutes*   *Servings: 1*

In a medium saucepan, combine 1 diced tomato, ¾ cup canned kidney beans, ½ cup canned black beans (rinsed and drained), ¼ cup chopped yellow or white onion, 1 rib chopped celery, 3 sliced baby carrots, ½ teaspoon each chili powder and cumin, 1 cup low-sodium chicken broth, and 1 tablespoon balsamic vinegar. Stir well and bring to a boil, then turn down the heat and simmer for 20 minutes. Add water during cooking, if needed. Top your hot soup with 1 tablespoon Parmesan cheese.

Taco Salad

Prep: 11 minutes   *Cook: 9 minutes*   *Servings: 1*

Lightly coat a skillet with olive oil cooking spray and warm over low to medium heat. Add 3 ounces ground turkey breast meat and sprinkle with ⅛ teaspoon each dried cumin and chili powder. Stir until cooked through, about 7 to 9 minutes. Make a salad with 2 cups romaine lettuce, ½ cup salsa, ½ cup diced red bell pepper, the cooked turkey breast, 2 tablespoons light salad dressing such as ranch (about 80 calories' worth of dressing), 2 tablespoons shredded reduced-fat Cheddar cheese, ⅓ cup reduced-fat feta cheese, and ½ ounce baked tortilla chips (about 9 crumbled chips).

Tomato Couscous with Spicy Grilled Eggplant

Prep: 11 minutes   *Cook: 30 minutes*   *Servings: 1*

Preheat the oven to 350°F. Prepare 1 cup cooked couscous and toss with 1 teaspoon extra-virgin olive oil, 1 tablespoon Parmesan cheese, ¼ teaspoon dried basil, 2 tablespoons sliced black olives, 1 minced garlic clove, and 1 diced tomato. Lightly coat a baking sheet with olive oil cooking spray, slice ½ of a small eggplant, and spread on the tray. Drizzle with 2 teaspoons extra-virgin olive oil and sprinkle with 1 tablespoon Parmesan cheese; ¼ teaspoon each black pepper, sage, and parsley; and ⅛ teaspoon cayenne pepper and bake for 17 to 20 minutes.

Peach and Cottage Cheese Wrap

Prep: 4 minutes   *Servings: 1*

Lay out 1 whole wheat soft tortilla and fill with ¼ cup 1% or fat-free cottage cheese and 1 sliced peach. Serve with 6 ounces fat-free Stonyfield Farm Peach, Raspberry, Strawberry, French Vanilla, Apricot-Mango, Berry Bash, Black Cherry, or Blueberry yogurt.

Grilled Vegetable Sandwich

Prep: 11 minutes   *Cook: 8 minutes*   *Servings: 1*

Lightly coat a skillet with olive oil cooking spray and heat over low to medium heat. Add ½ of a sliced green pepper, ¼ cup sliced mushrooms, 1 diced tomato, ¼ teaspoon each dried basil and dried oregano, and 1 teaspoon extra-virgin olive oil and sauté for 5 to 6 minutes, stirring occasionally. Open and toast (if desired) 1 whole wheat roll and top with 1 slice light Swiss cheese and the grilled vegetables. Serve with 1 sliced orange.

Dijon Chicken with Parmesan Vegetables

Prep: 13 minutes   *Cook: 35 minutes*   *Servings: 1*

Preheat the oven to 350°F. Lightly coat a baking dish with olive oil cooking spray. Add a 4-ounce raw chicken breast and brush with 1 teaspoon Dijon mustard. Slice ¼ of an eggplant and 1 zucchini and add them around the chicken. Spray the vegetables with olive oil cooking spray, drizzle with 1 tablespoon extra-virgin olive oil, and sprinkle with ¼ teaspoon each thyme and black pepper. Sprinkle the chicken and vegetables with 2 tablespoons Parmesan cheese. Bake for 35 minutes, or until the chicken is cooked through. Serve with 1 sliced papaya.

KEEP-ON-LOSING CORE DIET RECIPES

Below you'll find the recipes you will use during the Keep-On-Losing Phase. As with phase 1, I've listed these meals in the order that you will use them in the meal plan. Enjoy!

DAY 15

Creamy Spinach Pasta

Prep: 4 minutes   *Cook: 12 minutes*   *Servings: 1*

Combine ½ cup cooked whole wheat pasta, any shape, in a microwave-safe bowl with 2 cups fresh spinach, ¾ cup fat-free ricotta cheese, 1 minced garlic clove, 2 teaspoons extra-virgin olive oil, and ¼ cup roasted red peppers from the jar chopped into tiny pieces. Stir to combine and heat in the microwave for 90 seconds to 2 minutes to warm, stirring once. Serve with 1 sliced mango or 125 calories of your favorite fruit.

DAY 15

Minestrone Soup and Bruschetta

Prep: 8 minutes   *Cook: 6 minutes*   *Servings: 1*

Have 1½ cups of minestrone soup such as Campbell's Healthy Request Minestrone Soup and top with ¼ cup shredded reduced-fat mozzarella cheese. Serve with 1 slice of quick bruschetta: Drizzle a slice of whole wheat bread with 2 teaspoons extra-virgin olive oil and top with 1 small chopped tomato, ¼ teaspoon dried basil, 1 teaspoon minced garlic clove, and 2 teaspoons Parmesan cheese. Bake for 4 minutes at 200°F or toast in the toaster oven.

DAY 16
French Toast

Prep: 14 minutes   *Cook: 12 minutes*   *Servings: 2*

In a medium bowl, whisk together 3 egg whites and ⅓ cup fat-free milk. Coat a large skillet with butter-flavored cooking spray and heat over low to medium heat. Add 1½ tablespoons light canola oil butter, and while it's melting, dip 3 slices of whole wheat bread into the egg mixture and then add to the skillet. Sprinkle the 3 slices with ½ teaspoon ground cinnamon. Turn the bread over and cook until the egg is set on both sides. Serve 1½ slices now; save 1½ slices for breakfast another day. Package the extra portion in a zipper-lock bag, and it will keep for 3 days in the refrigerator and up to 1 month in the freezer. Immediately before serving, top each serving with ½ cup frozen, unsweetened blueberries and 6 ounces fat-free Stonyfield Farm Peach, Raspberry, Strawberry, French Vanilla, Apricot-Mango, Berry Bash, Black Cherry, or Blueberry yogurt. Serve with 1 cup fat-free milk.

DAY 16
Just-Like-Chinese-Takeout

Prep: 8 minutes   *Cook: 15 minutes*   *Servings: 1*

Coat a skillet with plain cooking spray and 1 teaspoon sesame oil and heat over low to medium heat. Add 2 cups Chinese-style vegetables (bok choy, broccoli, carrots, water chestnuts) or any mixed vegetable and sauté for 2 to 3 minutes, stirring frequently. Add 1 teaspoon reduced-sodium soy sauce, 1 tablespoon rice vinegar, 1 tablespoon sesame seeds, ½ cup cooked brown rice, and 3 (heated) Boca Meatless Chik'n Nuggets or 1 Tyson Low-Fat Chicken Patty (chopped into small pieces). Sauté, stirring frequently, for another 2 minutes.

Applesauce Pancakes

Prep: 9 minutes   *Cook: 10 minutes*   *Servings: 2*

Coat a skillet with butter-flavored cooking spray and heat over low to medium heat. In a bowl, combine ½ cup whole wheat pancake mix with 1 egg white (or ⅛ cup egg substitute), ¼ cup plus 2 tablespoons fat-free milk, and ¼ cup applesauce. Pour ¼ cup batter for each pancake and flip when tops are covered with bubbles and the edges look cooked. Have 1 serving now and save 1 serving for breakfast another day. Package the extra portions in a zipper-lock bag, and they will keep for 3 days in the refrigerator and up to 1 month in the freezer. Immediately before serving, top each serving with ½ cup frozen, unsweetened blackberries and 3 ounces fat-free Stonyfield Farm Peach, Raspberry, Strawberry, French Vanilla, Apricot-Mango, Berry Bash, Black Cherry, or Blueberry yogurt (half of a 6-ounce container). Serve with 1 cup fat-free milk.

Artichoke Pizza

Prep: 7 minutes   *Cook: 12 minutes*   *Servings: 4*

Preheat the oven to 400°F. Lay out one 12" whole wheat thin pizza crust, such as Boboli 100% Whole Wheat Thin Crust, and layer with 1 cup fresh spinach, 10 marinated artichoke hearts, and ½ cup chopped red onion. Top with 1 ounce goat cheese and bake for 12 minutes. Serve ¼ of the pizza now and save the remainder in the refrigerator for up to 3 days or freeze for up to 1 month.

Southwestern Scrambled Eggs

Prep: 6 minutes   *Cook: 7 minutes*   *Servings: 1*

Coat a skillet with olive oil cooking spray and heat over low to medium. Add 2 lightly beaten egg whites mixed with 2 tablespoons fat-free milk and scramble for 4 to 6 minutes, or until the eggs are set. Open a 6" whole wheat pita and fill with the scrambled eggs and ½ cup salsa. Serve with ¾ cup strawberries and 1 cup fat-free milk mixed with 2 teaspoons flavored coffee creamer, heated on high in the microwave for 30 to 60 seconds.

Teriyaki Swordfish

Prep: 16 minutes   *Cook: 15 minutes*   *Servings: 1*

Preheat the oven to 350°F. Coat a baking dish with plain cooking spray. In a zipper-lock bag, add 1½ teaspoons reduced-sodium teriyaki sauce, 1 teaspoon sesame oil, ½ teaspoon grated orange peel, and ½ teaspoon minced garlic. Add a 3-ounce swordfish steak to the bag and let it marinate in the refrigerator for 10 minutes. Place the swordfish in the baking dish and bake for 15 minutes. Serve with 1½ cups romaine lettuce topped with ¼ cup grated carrots, ½ cup canned chickpeas (rinsed and drained), and 1 small chopped tomato. Top with 2 tablespoons light salad dressing (about 80 calories' worth).

Spinach Dip and Whole Wheat Crackers

Prep: 7 minutes   *Cook: 4 minutes*   *Servings: 1*

Combine 5 ounces frozen cut-leaf spinach, cooked and drained of excess water, with ½ cup fat-free sour cream, ½ teaspoon onion powder, and ¼ cup water chestnuts. Scoop the dip with 5 Ak-Mak brand crackers, 12 reduced-fat Triscuit crackers, or 200 calories of your favorite trans-free, whole wheat cracker.

Falafel

Prep: 11 minutes   *Cook: 9 minutes*   *Servings: 1*

Prepare 1 serving of falafel, such as Fantastic Foods Falafel Mix, using ¼ cup dry mix and 1 tablespoon canola oil. Fill a 6" whole wheat pita with ½ cup thinly sliced red pepper, a handful of romaine lettuce, and 1 sliced tomato. Mince both ¼ of a cucumber and 1 garlic clove and mix together with 6 ounces fat-free plain Greek yogurt. Top the falafel with the yogurt dressing.

Lemon and Dill Chicken with Caesar Salad

Prep: 40 minutes   *Cook: 11 minutes*   *Servings: 1*

In a zipper-lock bag, combine 2 tablespoons lemon juice and 1 teaspoon dried dill. Add a 4-ounce raw chicken breast to the bag and marinate in the refrigerator for 30 minutes to overnight. Coat a skillet with olive oil cooking spray and heat over low to medium heat. Add the chicken and cook on both sides for 7 to 9 minutes, or until cooked through. Make a side salad with 1½ cups romaine lettuce, 1 tablespoon Parmesan cheese, and home-made croutons. To make the croutons, toast 1 slice pumpernickel bread spread with 2 teaspoons light canola oil butter and sprinkled with ¼ teaspoon dried basil, then cut into squares. Top the salad with 2 tablespoons light Caesar dressing (or 80 calories' worth of your favorite dressing) and toss well. Serve with 1 plum.

Mesquite Chicken Salad

At Applebee's restaurant, order the Onion Soup au Gratin and the Mesquite Chicken Salad from the Weight Watchers menu. At TGIF, order a cup of French onion soup (or a vegetable-based soup) and the Santa Fe Chicken Salad (have half of this salad; split it with your dining partner). Elsewhere, order a cup of French onion soup and a Southwest-style chicken salad and leave off the cheese. The salad portions should be about 4 ounces of chicken breast (the size of a bar of soap) and ½ cup each of corn, black beans, tomatoes, and peppers (each about the size of a baseball). Ask for a light dressing on the side and use 2 tablespoons.

DAY 22
Idaho Potato and Eggs

Prep: 12 minutes   *Cook: 11 minutes*   *Servings: 1*

Pierce a 3-ounce potato with a fork a few times and heat in the microwave on high for 3 to 4 minutes. Allow the potato to cool, then chop it. Coat a skillet with olive oil cooking spray and heat over low to medium heat. Whisk together 3 egg whites and 3 tablespoons fat-free milk and add to skillet with the potato and 1 cup fresh spinach leaves. Sprinkle with ⅛ teaspoon each onion powder and black pepper. Scramble about 4 to 6 minutes, or until the eggs are set. Serve with 1 cup fat-free milk and 1 sliced kiwifruit.

DAY 22
Cheese Quesadilla

Prep: 7 minutes   *Cook: 6 minutes*   *Servings: 1*

Preheat the oven to 350°F. On a 10" square of aluminum foil, lay an 8" whole wheat tortilla and top with ½ cup canned kidney beans (rinsed and drained), 2 tablespoons sliced black olives, ¼ cup diced green pepper, and 3 tablespoons shredded reduced-fat Cheddar cheese. Roll up the tortilla, wrap with the foil, and heat for 6 minutes. Serve with 1 cup fat-free milk.

Fruit Shake

Prep: 4 minutes   *Servings: 1*

In a blender, combine 2 ounces tofu (with calcium sulfate); 1 large sliced peach; 6 ounces fat-free Stonyfield Farm Peach, Raspberry, Strawberry, French Vanilla, Apricot-Mango, Berry Bash, Black Cherry, or Blueberry yogurt; 4 tablespoons calcium-fortified orange juice; ½ cup fat-free milk; 1 cup raspberries; and ½ teaspoon vanilla extract. Blend until smooth.

Beef and Brown Rice

Prep: 12 minutes   *Cook: 19 minutes*   *Servings: 1*

Combine 4 ounces round, sirloin, or flank steak cut into 1" pieces with ¼ cup dry brown rice; ½ cup reduced-fat, reduced-sodium cream of mushroom soup such as Campbell's Healthy Request; ¼ cup water; ½ cup sliced mushrooms; and 1 medium chopped carrot. Mix well, cover, and cook in the slow cooker on low for 7 to 8 hours.

Variation: To cook on the stovetop, prepare ½ cup cooked brown rice. Coat a pan with cooking spray and heat over low to medium heat and brown the sirloin for 6 to 7 minutes, turning once. Turn down to simmer and add the brown rice with the vegetables and soup and simmer for 2 minutes, or until warmed through.

Orzo Carrot Pecan Salad

Prep: 9 minutes   *Cook: 10 minutes*   *Servings: 1*

Prepare ½ ounce dry orzo with 3 cups water. Three minutes short of the end time for cooking, add ½ cup shredded carrot to the orzo and water and continue to boil for 3 minutes. Drain the orzo and carrots in a colander. Combine 1 sliced banana with the orzo and carrots and add 2 tablespoons chopped pecans, 1 teaspoon brown sugar, and 1 tablespoon light canola oil butter. Serve with 1 cup fat-free milk.

White Bean and Tuna Salad

Prep: 9 minutes   *Servings: 1*

Combine 2 cups mixed greens with 1 chopped red tomato and 1 cup fresh broccoli florets. Top with ½ cup canned white cannellini beans (rinsed and drained), 3 ounces chunk light tuna packed in water (rinsed and drained), 1 tablespoon rice vinegar, 1 tablespoon extra-virgin olive oil, ½ grapefruit (peeled and sectioned), and 1 tablespoon capers (if desired) and toss well.

Quick Peach Cobbler

Prep: 6 minutes   *Cook: 4 minutes*   *Servings: 1*

In a microwave-safe bowl, combine 1 sliced fresh peach, ½ cup low-fat granola, 2 tablespoons calcium-fortified orange juice, and 1 teaspoon grated orange peel. Heat on high in the microwave for 3 minutes, let stand for 1 minute, then top with 1 tablespoon fat-free sour cream and 1 tablespoon toasted slivered almonds.

Waldorf Salad

Prep: 4 minutes   *Servings: 1*

In a medium bowl, mix 2 cups spring mix greens with 1 small chopped apple, 2 ribs chopped celery, ½ cup grapes, ¼ of a 6-ounce container of fat-free Stonyfield Farm Lotsa Lemon yogurt, and 10 walnut halves. Serve with the remaining yogurt on the side.

Sesame Chicken

Prep: 11 minutes　　　*Cook: 45 minutes*　　　*Servings: 1*

Preheat the oven to 400°F. Coat a small baking dish with plain cooking spray and add 2 teaspoons olive oil to the pan. In a zipper-lock bag, combine 1 tablespoon sesame seeds, 1 tablespoon whole wheat flour, and ⅛ teaspoon black pepper. Add a 4-ounce raw chicken breast to the bag and shake to coat. Lay the chicken breast in the baking dish and bake for 35 minutes. Serve with ½ cup cooked brown rice mixed with 1 teaspoon olive oil, 1 diced tomato, 2 teaspoons balsamic vinegar, and a sprinkle of black pepper.

DAY 25
Salmon Caesar Salad

At a family-style restaurant, order the salmon Caesar salad with light dressing and the Parmesan cheese on the side, using about a palm-size amount of salmon and about a tennis-ball-size amount of croutons. Dip your fork in the dressing with each forkful of salad; this will keep your portion of salad dressing under 2 tablespoons. Sprinkle on about a ping-pong-ball size amount of Parmesan cheese. Serve with a side of a 3"-diameter crusty whole wheat or French roll.

DAY 25
Pasta with Goat Cheese

Prep: 9 minutes　　　*Cook: 16 minutes*　　　*Servings: 1*

Coat a skillet with olive oil cooking spray, add 1 tablespoon extra-virgin olive oil, and heat over medium. Add 1 cup broccoli florets and ½ cup sliced orange bell pepper and cook for 4 minutes, stirring constantly. Turn down the heat to low and add 1 cup cooked whole wheat pasta, any shape, and toss with 1½ teaspoons Dijon mustard, 1 tablespoon lemon juice, 1 teaspoon minced garlic, 1 tablespoon Parmesan cheese, and 1 ounce soft goat cheese (break into small pieces). Cook for another minute, stirring constantly, and serve warm.

Spinach and Feta Pizza

Prep: 6 minutes   *Cook: 12 minutes*   *Servings: 4*

Preheat the oven to 400°F. Lay out one 12" whole wheat thin pizza crust such as Boboli 100% Whole Wheat Thin Crust and layer with 1 tablespoon extra-virgin olive oil, 2 cups fresh spinach (tear into small pieces), and 3 ounces crumbled feta cheese. Bake for 12 minutes. Eat ¼ of the pizza, splitting the remainder with your family or saving it in the refrigerator for up to 3 days or in the freezer for up to 1 month. Eat with 1 sliced orange.

DAY 27
Big Chef Salad

Prep: 9 minutes   *Cook: 2 minutes*   *Servings: 1*

Mix together 1 cup baby spinach leaves and 1 cup romaine lettuce, sprinkle with ⅓ cup shredded reduced-fat mozzarella cheese and 2 ounces deli ham sliced into strips, and toss with 2 tablespoons light ranch dressing (or 80 calories of your favorite dressing) and homemade croutons. To make the croutons, toast 1 slice whole wheat bread spread with 1 tablespoon light canola oil butter and sprinkled with ¼ teaspoon dried basil, then cut into squares.

DAY 27
Apricot Fish with Baked Sweet Potato Fries

Prep: 22 minutes   *Cook: 30 minutes*   *Servings: 1*

Preheat the oven to 350°F. Coat a baking dish with olive oil cooking spray. In a zipper-lock bag, add 1 teaspoon extra-virgin olive oil, 2 tablespoons apricot preserves, 1 tablespoon lemon juice, and ½ teaspoon cooking sherry. Add a 4-ounce fillet of white fish such as tilefish or snapper to the bag and allow to marinate in the refrigerator for 10 minutes. In the meantime, slice a 4-ounce sweet potato into strips and place in the baking dish, drizzle with 2 teaspoons extra-virgin olive oil, and sprinkle with ½ teaspoon each black pepper and paprika. Bake for 15 minutes, then add the fish, and return to the oven for 15 minutes.

Tuna with Parmesan Spinach

Prep: 8 minutes *Cook: 3 minutes* *Servings: 1*

Microwave a 9-ounce bag of fresh baby spinach on high for 2 minutes. Carefully remove the hot spinach from the bag and fork out into a microwave-safe bowl. Add 4 ounces chunk light tuna packed in water (rinsed and drained) and 2 teaspoons extra-virgin olive oil and mix together lightly. Sprinkle with 2 tablespoons Parmesan cheese. Microwave on high for 30 to 45 seconds, until the cheese begins to melt. Serve with 6 ounces fat-free Stonyfield Farm French Vanilla yogurt.

Grilled Chicken with Arugula Salad and Maple Corn

Prep: 25 minutes *Cook: 33 minutes* *Servings: 1*

Preheat the grill for 10 minutes. Marinate a 3-ounce raw chicken breast in a zipper-lock bag with 1 teaspoon olive oil and 1 tablespoon lemon juice and sprinkle with black pepper. In the meantime, unwrap the husks on the corn, remove the silks, and rewrap the corn with the husks. Soak the corn (with husks on) in water for 15 minutes. Open the husks, brush each ear of corn with 2 teaspoons maple syrup, spread each ear with 2 teaspoons light butter, and rewrap the husks. Grill the corn for 4 minutes, turn once, and grill for another 4 minutes. Then place the corn on a higher shelf in the grill, close the grill, and allow it to roast for 15 minutes. Grill the chicken breast for 8 to 10 minutes. Unwrap the husks from the corn right before serving. Serve with 2 cups of arugula leaves topped with balsamic vinegar.

INDEX

Boldface page references indicate photographs.

Underscored references indicate boxed text.

Tuna
Tuna with Parmesan Spinach, 282
White Bean and Tuna Salad, 279
Turkey
Parmesan Turkey Pasta with Vegetables, 261
Turkey Tahini Sandwich, 228

U

Uppercuts, 170, **170**

V

Vegetables
Bell Pepper and Carrots with Onion Dip, 265
benefits of, 53
Dijon Chicken with Parmesan Vegetables, 271
dips for, 237
frozen, 247
Grilled Vegetable Sandwich, 271
organic, 236
Parmesan Turkey Pasta with Vegetables, 261
Salmon and Veggies with Spicy Ranch Sauce, 267
Venison meat, 246

W

Waffle with Ricotta Topping, 237
Waistbands, tight, 228
Waistline chop on the ball, 163, **163**
Waistline slimmer, 161, **161**
Waist measurement, 20, 32
Waist-to-hip ratio (WHR), 32–33
Walking
dog, 221
instead of driving, 227, 254
with music, 249
postpregnancy, 66
power, 248
while on phone, 235
Warmup standing side stretch, 128, **128,** 169, **169**

Warmup standing stretch, 127, **127,** 168, **168**
Warrior II, 49, **49**
Water, 234
Weight, body
fluid, <u>231</u>
weekly weigh-in, 208, 255
Weight training, 14, 74, 76
Whole grains, 214
WHR, 32–33
Worrying, 238
Wraps
Chunky Peanut Wrap, 246
Fruit and Cheese Tortilla Wrap, 235
Peach and Cottage Cheese Wrap, 271

Y

Yoga
breathing technique, 216
classes, 255
Yoga bridge stretch, 166, **166**
Yogurt
Berry Chocolate, 244
sugar in, 234